Affiliated with European Pancreatic Club (EPC)

Digestion

International Journal of Gastroenterology

Founded as 'Archiv für Verdauungskrankheiten' 1895 by I. Boas
Continued as 'Gastroenterologia' 1939–1967
Former Editors: P. Morawitz (1934–1936), R. Staehelin (1937–1943), A. Hurst (1940–1945), W. Löffler (1943–1961), Th.C. Hunt (1947–1967), N. Henning (1953–1962), B. Ihre (1953–1967), H. Bartelheimer (1963–1967), M. Demole (1963–1971), H. Kapp (1968–1970), R. Lambert (1972–1978), W. Creutzfeldt (1979–1992)

KARGER

Printed in Switzerland
on acid-free paper by
Reinhardt Druck, Basel

Appears bimonthly:
1 volume per year
(6 issues)

Guidelines for Authors

Digestion

Submission

'Digestion' invites papers covering investigative physiology in humans and animals, metabolic studies, and clinical work on etiology, diagnosis, and therapy of human diseases. Only original papers written in English are considered and should be sent to:

R. Arnold, MD, FRCP
Professor of Internal Medicine
Department of Internal Medicine
Philipps University
Baldingerstrasse
D–35033 Marburg (Germany)
Telephone +49 6421 286460
Telefax +49 6421 288922

Manuscripts should be submitted in four copies (with four sets of original illustrations, typewritten double-spaced on one side of the paper, with a wide margin. **The names, addresses and fax numbers of four experts in the appropriate area of research should accompany each manuscript. Selected scientist(s) will be invited to act as referee(s).**

Conditions

All manuscripts are subject to editorial review. Manuscripts are received with the explicit understanding that they are not under simultaneous consideration by any other publication. Submission of an article for publication implies the transfer of the copyright from the author to the publisher upon acceptance. Accepted papers become the permanent property of 'Digestion' and may not be reproduced by any means, in whole or in part, without the written consent of the publisher. It is the author's responsibility to obtain permission to reproduce illustrations, tables, etc. from other publications.

Special Requirements

1. Investigations Involving Human Subjects: 'Digestion' requires that investigations performed on human subjects have the prior approval of the institutional committee on human experimentation. Authors are required to submit a signed statement as to the date and details of the appropriate review. In countries where such mechanisms for approval do not exist, authors are required to submit a signed declaration that the research was carried out in accordance with the Helsinki Declaration. A similar assurance is required to document that animal experimentation was performed under appropriate circumstances.

2. Statement for Authors Submitting Original Research or Case Reports: 'The enclosed manuscript ... (Title)... has been approved by me as well as by the responsible authorities at the institute where the work has been carried out.
I certify that none of the material in this manuscript has been published previously in any form and that none of this material is currently under consideration for publication elsewhere. This includes symposia and proceedings of meetings and preliminary publications of any kind except an abstract of 400 words or less.'
(To be signed by *all* authors)

3. The undersigned also confirm that they qualify for (co-) authorship according to the 'Uniform Requirements for Manuscripts' published in the guidelines of the 'International Committee of Medical Journal Editors' in 1988 as follows: Authorship credit should be based only on substantial contributions to (a) conception and design, or analysis and interpretation of data; (b) drafting the article or revising it critically for important intellectual content; and on (c) final approval of the version to be published. Conditions (a), (b), and (c) must all be met. Participation solely in the acquisition of funding or the collection of data does not justify authorship. General supervision of the research group is also not sufficient for authorship. Any part of an article critical to its main conclusions must be the responsibility of at least one author. Persons who have contributed intellectually to the article but whose contributions do not justify authorship may be named and their particular contribution described in the section 'Acknowledgements'. Such persons must give their permission to be named.

Arrangement

Title page: The first page of each paper should indicate the title (main title underlined), the authors' names, and the institute where the work was conducted. A short title for use as running head as well as the full address of the author to whom correspondence should be sent are also required.

Full address: The exact postal address complete with postal code must be given at the bottom of the title page. Please also supply phone and fax numbers, as well as your e-mail address.

Key words: For indexing purposes, a list of 3–10 key words in English is essential.

Abstract: Each paper needs an abstract of up to 200 words. It should be organized as follows:

Background/Aims:	What is the major problem that prompted the study?
Methods:	How was the study done?
Results:	Most important findings?
Conclusion:	Most important conclusion?

Small type: Paragraphs which can or must be set in smaller type (case histories, test methods, etc.) should be indicated with a 'p' (petit) in the margin on the left-hand side.

Footnotes: Avoid footnotes. When essential, they are numbered consecutively and typed at the foot of the appropriate page.

Tables and illustrations: Tables and illustrations (both numbered in Arabic numerals) should be prepared on separate sheets. Tables require a heading and figures a legend, also prepared on a separate sheet. For the reproduction of illustrations, only good drawings and original photographs can be accepted; negatives or photocopies cannot be used. Due to technical reasons, figures with a screen background should not be submitted. When possible, group several illustrations on one block for reproduction (max. size 181 × 223 mm) or provide crop marks. On the back of each illustration, indicate its number, the author's name, and 'top' with a soft pencil.

Color illustrations: Up to 6 color illustrations per page can be integrated with the text at the reduced price of CHF 660.– / USD 545.00 per page. Color illustrations are reproduced at the author's expense.

References: In the text identify references by Arabic numerals [in square brackets]. Material submitted for publication but not yet accepted should be noted as 'unpublished data' and not be included in the reference list. The list of references should include only those publications which are cited in the text. Do not alphabetize; number references in the order in which they are first mentioned in the text. The surnames of the authors followed by initials should be given. There should be no punctuation other than a comma to separate the authors. Cite all authors, 'et al.' is not sufficient. Abbreviate journal names according to the Index Medicus system. (Also see International Committee of Medical Journal Editors: Uniform requirements for manuscripts submitted to biomedical journals. Br Med J 1988;296:401–405.)

Examples
(a) Papers published in periodicals: Sun J, Koto H, Chung KF: Interaction of ozone and allergen challenges on bronchial responsiveness and inflammation in sensitised guinea pigs. Int Arch Allergy Immunol 1997;112:191–195.
(b) Monographs: Matthews DE, Farewell VT: Using and Understanding Medical Statistics, ed 3, revised. Basel, Karger, 1996.
(c) Edited books: Parren PWHI, Burton DR: Antibodies against HIV-1 from phage display libraries: Mapping of an immune response and progress towards antiviral immunotherapy; in Capra JD (ed): Antibody Engineering. Chem Immunol. Basel, Karger, 1997, vol 65, pp 18–56.

Page charges

There is no page charge for papers of 3 or fewer printed pages (including tables, illustrations and references). Each additional complete or partial page is charged to the author at CHF 275.– / USD 196.00. The allotted size of a paper is equal to approx. 10 manuscript pages (including tables, illustrations and references). The inability to pay the additional page charge will not prejudice publication of the paper. This will be decided by the Editor.

Galley proofs

Unless indicated otherwise, galley proofs are sent to the first-named author and should be returned with the least possible delay. Alterations made in galley proofs, other than the correction of printer's errors, are charged to the author. No page proofs are supplied.

Reprints

Order forms and a price list are sent with the galley proofs. Orders submitted after the issue is printed are subject to considerably higher prices.

KARGER
Fax + 41 61 306 12 34
E-Mail karger@karger.ch
www.karger.com

The Guidelines for Authors are available at:
www.karger.com/journals/dig/dig_gl.htm

Digestion

General Information

Publication data: 'Digestion' is published 6 times a year. Volume 60 with 6 issues appears in 1999.

Subscription rates: Subscriptions run for a full calendar year. Prices are given per volume.
Personal subscription:
Subscription + postage and handling
CHF 189.60 + CHF 23.50 Europe
CHF 189.60 + CHF 35.50 Overseas
USD 149.00 + USD 23.50
(Must be in the name of, billed to, and paid by an individual. Order must be marked 'personal subscription'.)
Institutional subscription:
Subscription + postage and handling
CHF 948.– + CHF 29.40 Europe
CHF 948.– + CHF 44.40 Overseas
USD 745.00 + USD 29.40
Airmail postage: CHF 36.–, USD 30.00.
(Extra per volume.)

Microforms: Please direct all enquiries and orders to: University Microfilms Inc.
300 North Zeeb Road, P.O. Box 1346
Ann Arbor, MI 48106-1346 (USA)

Subscription orders: Orders can be placed at agencies, bookstores, directly with the Publisher
S. Karger AG, P.O. Box,
CH–4009 Basel (Switzerland)
or with any of the following distributors:
Deutschland: S. Karger GmbH, Postfach
D–79095 Freiburg
France: Librairie Luginbühl
36, bd de Latour-Maubourg, F–75007 Paris
Great Britain, Ireland: S. Karger Publishers
58 Grove Hill Road
Tunbridge Wells, Kent TN1 1SP
USA: S. Karger Publishers, Inc.
26 West Avon Road, P.O. Box 529
Farmington, CT 06085
India, Bangladesh, Sri Lanka:
S. Karger India Subscription Agency
B–5/132 Safdarjung Enclave
New Delhi-110029
Japan: Katakura Libri, Inc.
2F, Marushima Bldg, 4-6-17, Yushima,
Bunkyo-ku, Tokyo 113-0034

Change of address: Both old and new address should be sent to the subscription source.

Single issues and back volumes: Information can be obtained through the Publisher.

Advertising: Correspondence and rate requests should be addressed to the Publisher.

Bibliographic indices: This journal is regularly listed in bibliographic services, including *Current Contents®*.

Copying: This journal has been registered with the Copyright Clearance Center (CCC), as indicated by the code appearing on the first page of each article.
For readers in the US, this code signals consent for copying of articles for personal or internal use, or for the personal or internal use of specific clients, provided that the stated fee is paid per copy directly to
Copyright Clearance Center Inc.
222 Rosewood Drive
Danvers, MA 01923 (USA)
A copy of the first page of the article must accompany payment. Consent does not extend to copying for general distribution, for promotion, for creating new works, or for resale. In these cases, specific written permission must be obtained from the copyright owner,
S. Karger AG,
P.O. Box, CH–4009 Basel (Switzerland).

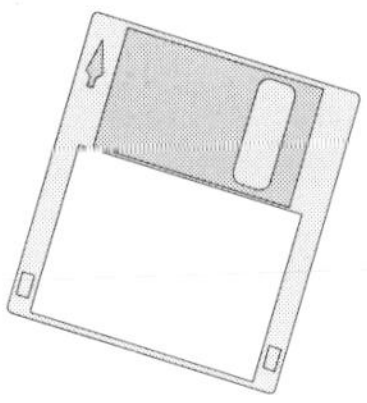

Disk Submission

A **comprehensive version** of these guidelines for the **submission of manuscripts and illustrations on disk** can be accessed online under **www.karger.com/journals/disksub.htm** or requested as a leaflet from the editorial department.

Please follow the general rules on style and arrangement in the **"Guidelines for Authors"** of the journal. Submit a **double-spaced printout** of your manuscript matching the file on disk exactly.

Technical Information
Store only data pertinent to this manuscript. Include your fonts (screen and printer fonts for Macintosh).
For a **text only** manuscript, use a 3.5 inch disk. For **text and illustrations,** use 3.5 or 5.25 Magneto Optical Disc; CD-ROM (DOS or hybrid); iomage Zip/DOS (100 MB), or 44 MB, 88 MB or 200 MB SyQuest. Compress extensive data using ZIP format.

Data Description
Label your disk with the **title of the journal or book** for which it is submitted; a **short version** of the paper's title; your **name,** postal and e-mail address, fax and phone number; **hard and software** used, including the version; and the **complete list of the file names.** File names consist of eight characters before the dot identifying the file and three characters after the dot identifying the application.

Text and Format
The **preferred word-processing package is MS-Word.** Other commonly used PC text programs and ASCII formats are accepted.
Update your data when you revise subsequent to the reviewer's or editor's decision and mark revisions clearly. Manuscripts accepted for publication are subject to **copy editing:** changes and/or questions will be marked in the manuscript, which will be returned to you with your disk and the galley proofs for checking.
Enter your text continuously flush left. Do not use any layout functions. Do not split words at the end of a line. **Do not use indentations.** Use a blank line before and a hard return at the end of paragraphs.
Arrange headings flush left. Insert only **one space after punctuation marks.** Insert Greek letters, mathematical symbols etc. with your word-processing program. Use **boldface and italics** as well as sub- and superscript where appropriate.
Tables are part of the text and should be placed at the end of the text file. Separate the individual parts of a table by lines. Use the tabulator instead of spaces. Format operation data on one line in the same column. **Legends to illustrations are part of the text** and should also be listed at the end of the text file.

Illustrations
Store illustrations as separate files: do not embed them in your text. Export **line drawings/vector graphics** as TIF, EPS or WMF format. Use Photoshop for processing and retouching **scanned halftone images.** Save the original scan and the processed version. Export **black and white or color images** as TIF or EPS format in their anticipated size in print.
For detailed information on how to submit illustration data on disk please consult the leaflet or **www.karger.com/journals/disksub.htm.**

KARGER

Fax + 41 61 306 12 34
E-Mail karger@karger.ch
www.karger.ch

The Journal Home Page is available at:
www.karger.com/journals/dig

KI 98 DISK

Digestion

Role of Somatostatin-Analogues in Gastrointestinal Diseases

Editors
Markus W. Büchler, Bern
Christoph Beglinger, Basel

9 figures, and 28 tables, 1999

KARGER
Basel · Freiburg · Paris · London · New York ·
New Delhi · Bangkok · Singapore · Tokyo · Sydney

S. Karger
Medical and Scientific Publishers
Basel · Freiburg · Paris · London
New York · New Delhi · Bangkok
Singapore · Tokyo · Sydney

Drug Dosage
The authors and the publisher have exerted every effort to ensure that drug selection and dosage set forth in this text are in accord with current recommendations and practice at the time of publication. However, in view of ongoing research, changes in government regulation, and the constant flow of information relating to drug therapy and drug reactions, the reader is urged to check the package insert for each drug for any change in indications and dosage and for added warnings and precautions. This is particularly important when the recommended agent is a new and/or infrequently employed drug.

P.O. Box, CH–4009 Basel (Switzerland)
Printed in Switzerland on acid-free paper by
Reinhardt Druck, Basel
ISBN 3–8055–6878–9

KARGER

Fax + 41 61 306 12 34
E-Mail karger@karger.ch
www.karger.ch

Digestion

Vol. 60, Suppl. 2, 1999

Contents

KARGER

Fax+ 41 61 306 12 34
E-Mail karger@karger.ch
www.karger.com

Access to full text and tables of contents,
including tentative ones for forthcoming issues:
www.karger.com/journals/dig/dig_bk.htm

Editorial

Digestion

Digestion 1999;60(suppl 2):1

A Decade of Octreotide

Somatostatin, a peptide hormone initially isolated from ovine hypothalami, has been documented to inhibit the release of growth hormone. It soon became evident that this peptide was not only present in the brain but was widely distributed in the stomach, the gastrointestinal tract and the pancreas. By 1980, the gene encoding for prosomatostatin had been identified and it became evident that different molecular forms are present in the body. Later on, different receptors for somatostatin were identified and it became clear that the different molecular forms and the different receptors are part of a complicated control system which regulate a variety of body functions. Somatostatin molecules exert profound inhibitory functions, not only on growth hormone secretion but also on many gastrointestinal functions. These different effects form the basis for an enormous therapeutic potential of somatostatin in different diseases. The short half-life of natural somatostatin which necessitates a continuous intravenous infusion has made it difficult to transform the natural peptide into a successful drug. It was therefore a major step forward when a synthetic analogue of somatostatin, octreotide, was synthesized and became available for clinical use in the mid-eighties. For over a decade, subcutaneous octreotide has proven effective in the treatment of acromegaly and in several clinical areas relating to gastroenterology and digestive surgery. The ability of octreotide to control symptoms such as diarrhea or flush caused by gut-neuroendocrine tumors soon became evident. Subsequently, octreotide was used in other forms of secretory diarrhea (AIDS-related diarrhea, idiopathic diarrhea, diabetic diarrhea) but also in the management of pancreatic disorders (pancreatic fistulae, prevention of complications following pancreatic surgery). Somatostatin analogues including octreotide have been shown to reduce pressure in the splanchnic circulation, an effect that was exploited in the management of variceal and nonvariceal hemorrhages.

Despite a widespread therapeutic application, octreotide seems to be a safe drug free of major side effects. Most of the reported side effects are gastrointestinal in nature and include steatorrhea, bloating, minor nausea, gallstones and mild forms of glucose intolerance. Recently a new formulation of octreotide, octreotide LAR® (long-acting repeatable), was developed which enables once-a-month administration. Octreotide LAR® combines over a decade of proven benefits of the subcutaneous octreotide administration with a more convenient formulation for long-term treatment of a variety of diseases. Once-monthly administration should improve patient acceptability and compliance; it represents a significant advance in the management of a number of conditions associated with excessive peptide secretion (acromegaly, neuroendocrine tumors). There is no doubt that additional indications will emerge as investigations continue. Treatment of certain gastrointestinal cancers and prevention of variceal bleeding are two clinical areas which are currently under investigation. A decade of octreotide has been beneficial for many patients; hopefully many more will be able to take advantage of this fascinating peptide.

Bern and Basel
January 1999

Markus W. Büchler
Christoph Beglinger

KARGER

Fax +41 61 306 12 34
E-Mail karger@karger.ch
www.karger.ch

0012–2823/99/0608–0001$17.50/0

Accessible online at:
http//BioMedNet.com/karger

Digestion

Digestion 1999;60(suppl 2):2–8

Somatostatin and Octreotide: Physiological Background and Pharmacological Application

Christoph Beglinger Jürgen Drewe

Divisions of Gastroenterology and Pharmacology, University Hospital, Basel, Switzerland

Key Words
Biological Effects · Octreotide · Octreotide LAR

Introduction

Molecular Structures. The ubiquitous distribution of somatostatin both in the central nervous system and in the periphery indicates the involvement of this peptide in multiple biological functions. The name somatostatin is given to a family of peptides, the original member of which, somatostatin-14 (S-14), a tetradecapeptide, was first extracted and isolated from ovine hypothalami [1]. The molecule was shown to inhibit growth hormone (GH) release in vitro and, later on, also in vivo [2, 3]. A second molecular form of somatostatin was reported in 1980 [4]; somatostatin-28 (S-28) contains the amino acid sequence of S-14, N-terminally extended by 14 amino acid residues (table 1). Today it is clear that somatostatin is synthesized as a prohormone which undergoes tissue-specific processing to produce either S-14 or S-28 [4]. The biological significance of the two forms remains to be determined in detail; current thinking suggests that S-14 predominantly acts as a neuropeptide, wheras S-28 operates as a true circulating hormone [5, 6].

Distribution. Large amounts of somatostatin are found in the gastrointestinal tract and in the pancreas, including the autonomic nervous system and specific endocrine cells. In addition, somatostatin is localized in the central nervous and the peripheral nervous system [3, 4, 7]. Immunocytochemical studies demonstrate that S-14 is localized in the D cells of the pancreas, the stomach and duodenum, wheras S-28 is the predominant form lower down the gut [7–9]. In addition, the gut is innervated by extrinsic and intrinsic S-14-containing neurons, with the intrinsic neurons being present both in the submucosal and myenteric plexus.

Somatostatin Receptors (SSTR). Multiple subtypes of receptors have been proposed to exist that mediate the biological actions of S-14 and S-28. The existence of multiple somatostatin receptor subtypes has recently been confirmed by the cloning of five different somatostatin receptors [10]. The cloning of these five receptor subtypes has led to the development of subtype-selective agonists. These compounds are revealing distinct functions of the individual receptor subtype which eventually may have a variety of therapeutic applications.

Biological Effects of Somatostatin

Effects on Hypothalamic Functions. The hypothalamus plays a critical role in the communication between the brain and the body as it is the site where information from higher centers is integrated and transduced to the periphery via the neuroendocrine and autonomous nervous systems [4, 5, 11]. Not surprisingly, therefore, hypothalamic anatomy is complex. The hypothalamus is connected to the pituitary gland by the hypothalamic-hypophyseal stalk which consists of (1) a portal vein system which carries the hypothalamic neurosecretory hor-

KARGER
Fax +41 61 306 12 34
E-Mail karger@karger.ch
www.karger.ch

0012–2823/99/0608–0002$17.50/0

Accessible online at:
http//BioMedNet.com/karger

Prof. Christoph Beglinger
Division of Gastroenterology, University Hospital
CH–4031 Basel (Switzerland)
Tel. +41 61 2652525/ext 181 2102
Fax +41 61 2653847, E-Mail beglinger@tmr.ch

Table 1. Amino acid sequences of S-14, S-28 and the somatostatin analogue octreotide

S-14	H-Ala-Gly-Cys-Lys-Asn-Phe-Phe-Trp-Lys-Thr-Phe-Thr-Ser-Cys-OH
S-28	H-Ser-Ala-Asn-Ser-Asn-Pro-Ala-Met-Ala-Pro-Arg-Glu-Arg-Lys-Ala-Gly-Cys-Lys-Asn-Phe-Phe-Trp-Lys-Thr-Phe-Thr-Ser-Cys-OH
Octreotide	H-(*D*)Phe-Cys-Phe-(*D*)Trp-Lys-Thr-Cys-Thr(ol)

mones, and (2) the axons of the paraventricular and supraoptic nuclei which travel to the neurohypophysis where they secrete their hormones (vasopressin, oxytocin) directly into the general circulation [13]. The anterior pituitary gland consists of five major cell types which secrete GH, thyrotropin, adrenocorticotrophic hormone (and other peptides), prolactin and the gonadotrophins. These hormones act on various peripheral tissues and endocrine organs. The original concept proposed that the hypothalamus would contain one releasing factor for each anterior pituitary hormone. In the search for such a releasing factor which would stimulate GH secretion, it came as a surprise to find a potent inhibitory factor which was subsequently identified as somatostatin [1, 2]. Only years later, GH-releasing hormone was identified and characterized [4].

The regulation of GH secretion has recently been reviewed [4]. Somatostatin acts at the somatotroph cells in the anterior pituitary gland to inhibit the secretion, but not the synthesis, of GH. Studies with somatostatin analogues suggest a role for SSTR2 and SSTR5 subtypes in mediating the inhibitory effect of somatostatin.

Effect of Somatostatin on the Gastroenteropancreatic Endocrine System. The previously mentioned anatomical considerations explain how somatostatin can have multiple endocrine, paracrine and neurocrine functions in addition to its GH release-inhibiting effect. The effects of somatostatin in the gastrointestinal tract are summarized in table 2. Somatostatin in pancreatic islet cell function has been described in numerous publications; two reviews are given for further reading [5, 12]. Somatostatin has been shown to inhibit the secretion of insulin, of glucagon, and of somatostatin itself. Most experts accept the view that somatostatin acts primarily as a paracrine agent in the gastrointestinal tract. Evidence supporting the concept that S-28 acts as a true hormone in humans has been provided by Ensinck and coworkers [6, 13–15]. Several studies have documented a rise in S-28 after nutrient intake without changes in S-14 [13, 14, 16] with fat being the most potent secretagogue of S-28 secretion. S-28 at postprandial concentrations significantly inhibits first-phase insulin secretion implying that S-28 released by nutrients from the distal ileum travels to the pancreatic islets where it acts as a true hormone [6]. These results form the basis for the concept and rationale which has been called the 'decretin concept', a nutrient-stimulated inhibitor of insulin secretion [6]. S-14, on the other hand, can act as a paracrine agent within the pancreatic islets, wheras S-28 acts as a true hormone to modulate insulin secretion. The relevance of these findings to the understanding of the pathogenesis of diabetes mellitus has still not been determined.

Somatostatin exerts an extraordinary range of physiologic effects on the gut including suppression of digestive hormones (gastrin, cholecystokinin, secretin), of gastric acid secretion and exocrine pancreatic secretion, of intestinal secretions, of motor activity (gastric emptying, gallbladder contraction), of absorptive activity, and of blood flow. A majority of these effects are paracrine or neurocrine transduced by S-14; a particular example is the local feedback loop between gastrin and somatostain (fig. 1). Gastrin secretion is stimulated by intraluminal nutrient components and central cholinergic impulses, and inhibited by local somatostatin release. In turn, gastrin stimulates S-14 secretion from D cells which thus acts as a negative feedback loop. Cholinergic inputs also inhibit S-14 secretion and S-14 inhibits acetylcholine release [17]. Many additional factors participate in the regulation of gastrin release, an inhibitory effect on gastrin secretion is, however, dependent on local S-14 release. An inhibitory effect of elevated postprandial S-28 levels on pancreatic exocrine secretion has been reported [18] suggesting that the hormonal effects of circulating S-28 released during nutrient absorption are not restricted to the pancreatic B cells but can affect other targets/organs. Somatostatin has effects on motor activity of the stomach, intestine and gallbladder. The effects on gastric emptying and gallbladder contraction seem to be predominantly inhibitory actions. Many questions remain unanswered. It is still open, for example, which other functions are controlled by S-14 and/or S-28. A physiologic role can only be established when specific receptor antagonists

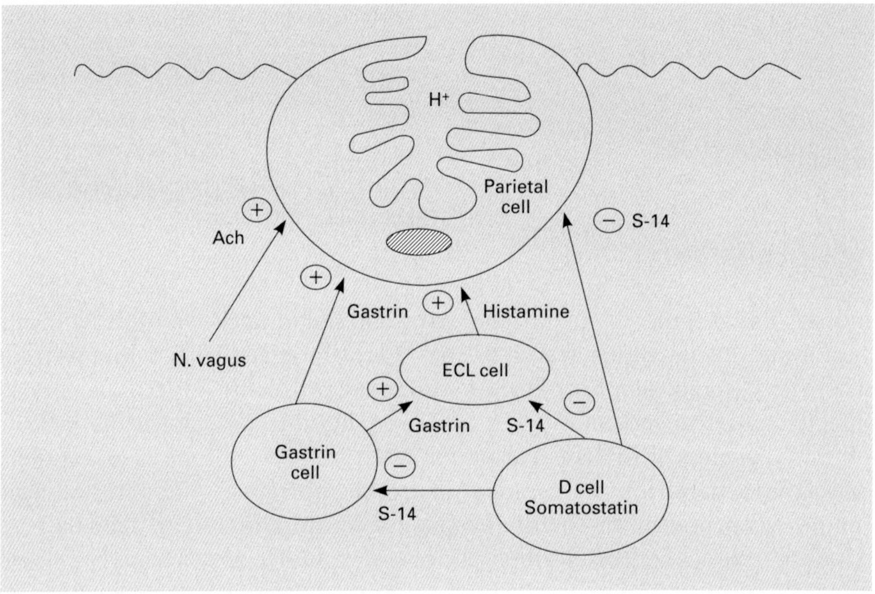

Fig. 1. Feedback loop between gastrin and somatostatin. For details see text.

Table 2. Biological effects of somatostatin on gastrointestinal functions

Inhibition of hormone secretion	Gastrin, cholecystokinin Secretin Insulin, glucagon, VIP
Inhibition of exocrine secretory responses	Gastric acid secretion Exocrine pancreatic secretion
Inhibition of motor activity	Gastric emptying Gallbladder contraction
Inhibition of nutrient absorption	
Stimulation of water and electrolyte absorption	
Inhibition of splanchnic/portal venous blood flow	

of the peptides become available. Finally, the expression pattern of the five different receptor subtypes is only partially defined. The existence of different receptor subtypes suggests however different physiologic functions. These observations furthermore imply the existence of a complex regulatory system which will only be unravelled when the exact roles of the subtypes expressed in the various tissues are defined.

Metabolism. The clearance rates of S-14 and S-28 in humans measured after exogenous infusion by radioimmunoassay have been found to be rapid. S-28 has a longer half-life and a slower clearance rate than S-14. The half-life of S-14 is about 1 min in humans, whereas the half-life of S-28 is about 3 times longer [15].

Octreotide

Pharmacokinetics. Based on the wide range of biological actions it was recognized that somatostatin has a potential for clinical applications. As pointed out before, natural somatostatin molecules are not ideal drugs. The short half-life of S-14 or S-28 necessitates a continuous intravenous infusion which is not suitable for long-term therapeutic use. Several synthetic somatostatin analogues have therefore been developed with improved metabolic stability and increased duration of action; some of these analogues have become available for clinical use (table 3). Amongst the different peptides, the octapeptides octreotide (Sandostatin®) and lanreotide (Somatuline®) have

Table 3. Synthetic somatostatin analogues in clinical use or development

Octreotide	Sandostatin®
Octreotide LAR	Sandostatin LAR®
Lanreotide	Somatuline®
Lanreotide SR	Somatuline SR®
Vapreotide	Octastatin®

Table 4. Pharmacokinetic characteristics of octreotide LAR after intramuscular administration (30 mg) [data modified from 22–24]

T_{max}, days	34±17
C_{max}, ng/l	1,935±1,430
Duration of plateau phase, days	19±10
Relative bioavailability, %	50

been most extensively investigated with octreotide receiving the major share of interest. Compared with natural somatostatin, octreotide shows a remarkable stability. This improved stability against proteolytic degradation, combined with a reduced hepatic clearance, is responsible for the dramatically improved elimination half-life. The pharmacokinetic properties of octreotide are summarized in table 4. The main characteristics are as follows: intravenous or subcutaneous applications of octreotide induce dose-dependent increases in plasma drug levels. Peak plasma concentrations after subcutaneous injections are reached within 30 min with a systemic bioavailability which is almost complete. The disposition half-life is more than 30 times the half-life of the natural peptide.

Pharmacodynamics. Octreotide preferentially binds to SSTR2, and to a lesser extent, to SSTR5 receptor subtypes. Based on this information, the biological effects can be predicted. Like natural somatostatin, octreotide exerts a potent inhibitory effect on GH secretion, but in addition, suppresses the secretion of a variety of peptides from the gastrointestinal-endocrine pancreatic (GEP) system. The main biological effects in the gut are similar to the effects summarized in table 2.

Octreotide inhibits most hormones of the gastrointestinal tract. Effective suppression of insulin and glucagon secretion can be achieved at very low plasma concentrations (fig. 2). Inhibition of cholecystokinin release is associated with a marked inhibition of gallbladder contraction (fig. 3) [12]; these effects may contribute to the development of gallstone disease, an undesired, potential adverse event of long-term therapy with somatostatin analogues (fig. 4). Octreotide and analogues are inhibitors of gastrin

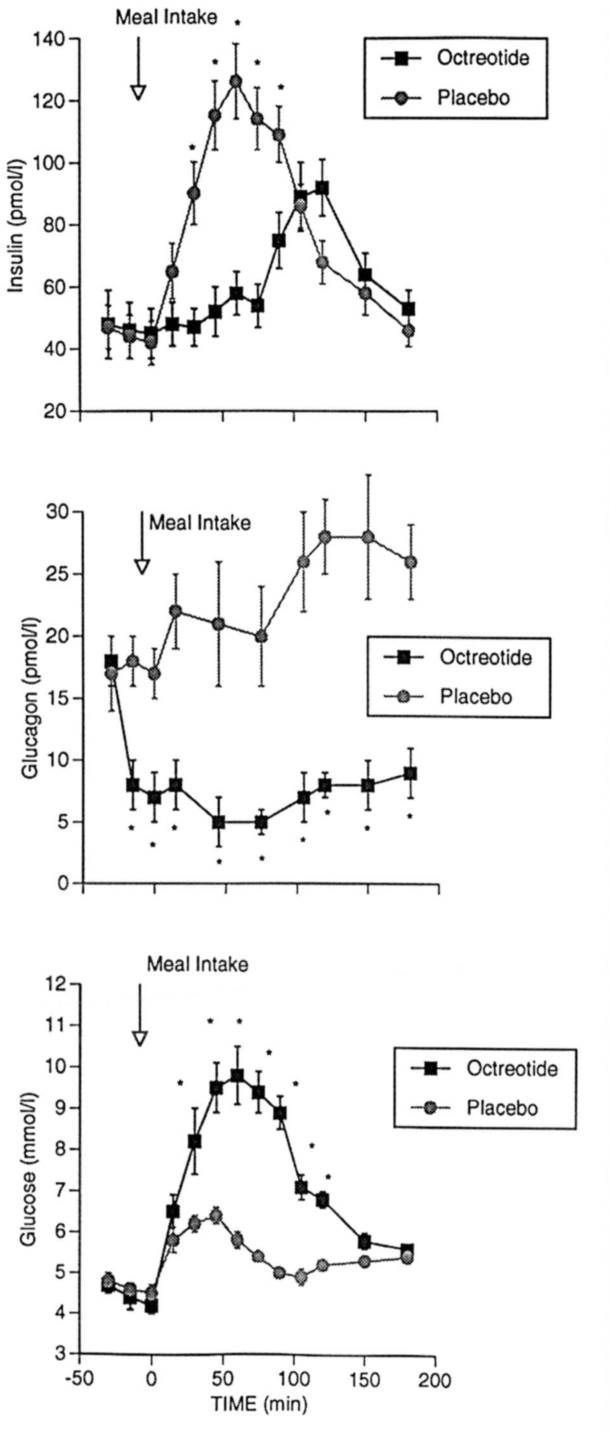

Fig. 2. Effect of octreotide (100 μg given as a single subcutaneous injection) on fasting and meal-stimulated plasma glucose, insulin and glucagon concentrations in 10 healthy male subjects. Data are mean±SEM. $*p<0.01$ vs. control [Drewe and Beglinger, unpubl. data].

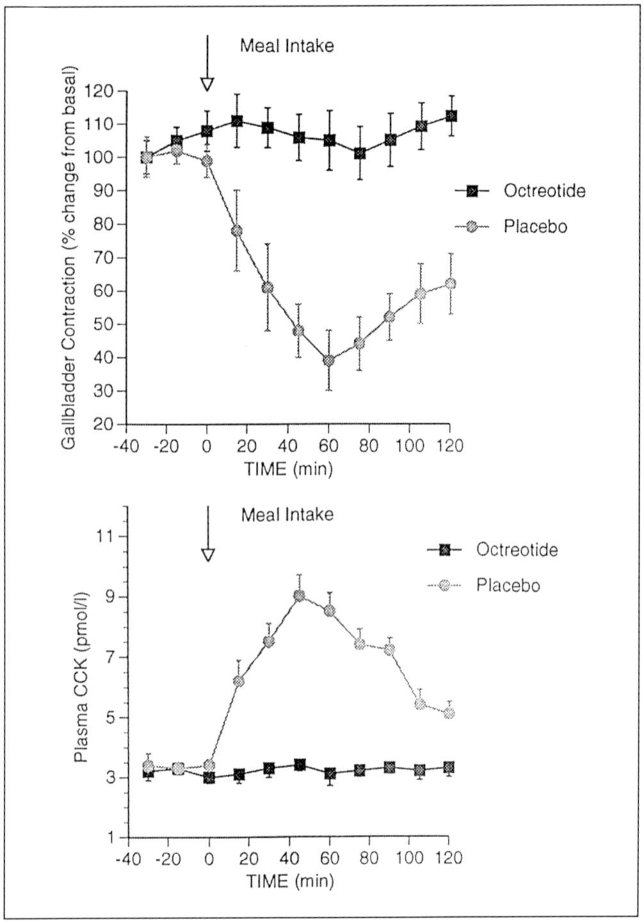

Fig. 3. Effect of octreotide (100 μg given as a single subcutaneous injection) on plasma cholecystokinin concentrations and gallbladder contraction in 10 healthy male subjects. Data are mean ± SEM. $*p<0.01$ vs. control [Drewe and Beglinger, unpubl. data].

release, but they exert additional effects on acid production by inhibiting histamine secretion from ECL cells and, perhaps, by directly inhibiting the parietal cell [17]. This inhibitory action decreases, however, with time. Octreotide also inhibits exocrine pancreatic secretory responses which form the basis for a therapeutic use of the compound in various pancreatic diseases [4, 19, 20]. Finally, octreotide and its analogues reduce postprandial splanchnic and portal venous blood flow, an effect which can be exploited in the treatment of esophageal varices [20, 21].

Octreotide Long-Acting Release

Octreotide has proved to be a valuable therapeutic tool to treat a variety of diseases. Long-term therapy requires, however, two to three daily injections which is inconvenient for the patient with potential effects on compliance. It was therefore most welcome that a new galenical formulation was developed for once-monthly intramuscular administration. The pharmacodynamic properties of the long-acting release (LAR) formulation of octreotide does not differ qualitatively from the original formulation of the subcutaneously administered drug. The various effects will therefore not be repeated here.

Pharmacokinetics. Octreotide LAR is based on a biodegradable polymer matrix (poly(*DL*-lactide-coglycolide glucose)) which releases the drug in a biphasic manner [22–24]. First, an initial peak in plasma octreotide concentrations is observed within 1 h after drug administration; this initial peak is due to drug release from the surface of the microspheres. This initial peak – less than 1% of the total amount of administered octreotide is released – is associated with a prolonged period of GH suppression (8–12 h) which is very similar to the suppression seen with a single subcutaneous injection of octreotide (fig. 5). Plasma drug concentrations decline after this initial peak and remain low for the next 7 days after the injection; a gradual increase is then observed and a plateau is reached at about day 14. This plateau remains stable for 4 weeks and then declines. In patients with acromegaly treated with octreotide LAR 20 mg, steady-state concentrations of the drug are reached after 3 intramuscular injections given at 4-week intervals. The optimal pharmacodynamic effect (suppression of GH secretion) is obtained when the plateau phase is reached. A dose-dependent increase in plateau concentrations was seen with increasing doses of octreotide LAR (dose proportionality). An advantage of the LAR formulation was a reduced fluctuation (25%) of peak and through octreotide concentrations compared to 200% fluctuations with intermittent subcutaneous injections [22–24]. In accordance with these observations, the variability in area under the curve (AUC) is less in patients receiving octreotide LAR (fluctuation 5–10%) compared to subcutaneous injections (about 40%).

Distribution and Elimination. Octreotide distributes mainly to the plasma and is approximatively 65% bound to proteins. 11–31% of the drug is eliminated unchanged in the urine, but the drug undergoes considerable hepatic extraction (30–40%). Clearance in chronic renal failure is slightly reduced; the effect of hepatic impairment on the clearance of octreotide has not been studied yet.

Tolerability. The database for adverse events after treatment with octreotide LAR is still rather small, because acromegaly and neuroendocrine tumors are rare

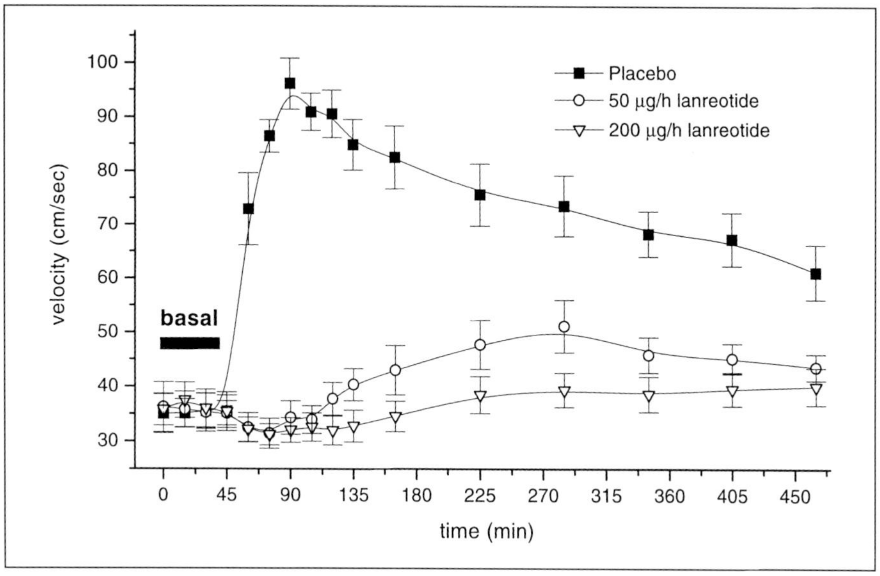

Fig. 4. Effect of increasing intravenous doses of the somatostatin analogue lanreotide on basal and meal-stimulated splanchnic blood flow in 8 healthy male subjects. Data are mean ± SEM. * $p < 0.01$ vs. control [modified from 21].

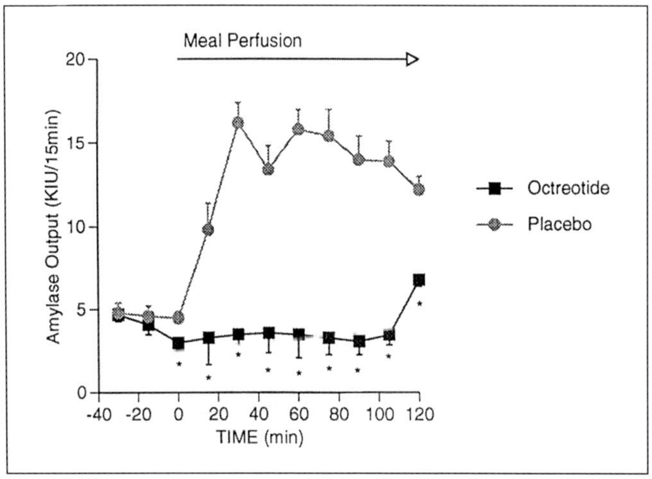

Fig. 5. Effect of octreotide (100 µg given as a single subcutaneous injection) on basal and meal-stimulated exocrine pancreatic secretory responses in 6 healthy male subjects. Data are mean ± SEM. * $p < 0.01$ vs. control [Beglinger, unpubl. data].

diseases. The main finding is, however, that the tolerability profile of this new formulation is very similar to that seen with subcutaneous injections. Gastrointestinal adverse events predominate: abdominal pain (sometimes in the form of cramps), flatulence and diarrhea were the most noted adverse events and were present in up to 50% of patients with acromegaly. The adverse events tended to be mild to moderate; they often disappeared within 1–4 days after injection; more importantly, the incidence decreased with long-term treatment. Steatorrhea is present with long-term octreotide treatment, but this is not associated with clinically significant malabsorption. The risk of gallstone development is increased with octreotide treatment, an effect which is believed to be related to the suppression of cholecystokinin release, inhibition of gallbladder motility and bile composition and secretion. Gallstones or biliary sludge develop in up to 50% of patients on long-term therapy, but most patients with octreotide-induced gallstones remain asymptomatic and do not require treatment. About 1% of patients become symptomatic and require medical intervention. Injection site events occurred in some patients (mild to moderate pain at the injection site; swelling and erythema).

Conclusions

Octreotide is a synthetic somatostatin analogue with prolonged biological activity as the molecule is protected against enzymatic degradation. The compound exhibits a broad spectrum of pharmacological actions similar to that of natural somatostatin. The most important effects for clinical application are: (1) inhibition of hormone production (insulin, glucagon, gastrin, VIP); (2) inhibition of exocrine pancreatic secretion; (3) inhibition of splanchic blood flow, and (4) promotion of water and electrolyte absorption.

Based on these biological effects, octreotide has been used to treat a variety of diseases in the gastrointestinal tract. Control of symptoms in patients with GEP tumors was one of the first indications for octreotide, but the molecule has been successfully used to treat other forms of noninfectious secretory diarrhea, but also to treat pancreatic diseases, fistulae and acute forms of gastrointestinal bleeding, especially variceal bleeding.

References

1 Krulich L, Dhariwal AP, McCann SM: Stimulatory and inhibitory effects of purified hypothalamic extracts on growth hormone release from rat pituitary in vitro. Endocrinology 1968;83:783–790.

2 Brazeau P, Vale W, Burgus R, et al: Hypothalamic polypeptide that inhibits the secretion of immunoreactive pituitary growth hormone. Science 1973;179:77–79.

3 Reichlin S: Somatostatin. N Engl J Med 1983;309:1495–1501.

4 Gillies G: Somatostatin: The neuroendocrine story. Trends Pharmacol Sci 1997;18:87–95.

5 Reichlin S: Secretion of somatostatin and its physiologic function. J Lab Clin Med 1987;109:320–326.

6 D'Alessio DA, Sieber C, Beglinger C, Ensinck JW: A physiologic role for somatostatin-28 as a regulator of insulin secretion. J Clin Invest 1989;84:857–862.

7 Baskin DG, Ensinck JW: Somatostatin in epithelial cells of intestinal mucosa is present primarily as somatostatin-28. Peptides 1984;5:615–621.

8 Alumets J, Sundler F, Hakanson B: Distribution, ontogeny and ultrastructure of somatostatin immunoreactive cells in the pancreas and gut. Cell Tissue Res 1977;185:465–479.

9 Larsson LI, Goltermann N, deMagistris JF, Rehfeld JF, Schwartz TW: Somatostatin cell processes and pathways for paracrine secretion. Science 1979;205:1393–1394.

10 Reisine T: Somatostatin receptors. Am J Physiol 1995;269:G813–G820.

11 Reichlin S: Somatostatin: Historical aspects. Scand J Gastroenterol Suppl 1986;119:1–10.

12 Bloom SR, Polak JM: Somatostatin. Br Med J 1987;295:288–290.

13 Ensinck JW, Laschansky EC, Vogel RE, Simonowitz DA, Roos BA, Francis BH: Circulating prosomatostatin-derived peptides. Differential responses to food ingestion. J Clin Invest 1989;83:1580–1589.

14 Ensinck JW, Vogel RE, Laschansky EC, Francis BH: Effect of ingested carbohydrate, fat, and protein on the release of somatostatin-28 in humans. Gastroenterology 1990;98:633–638.

15 Hildebrand P, Ensinck JW, Buettiker J, et al: Circulating somatostatin-28 is not a physiologic regulator of gastric acid production in man. Eur J Clin Invest 1994;24:50–56.

16 Shoelson SE, Polonsky KS, Nakabayashi T, Jaspan JB, Tager HS: Circulating forms of somatostatin-like immunoreactivity in human plasma. Am J Physiol 1986;250:E428–E434.

17 Walsh JH: Gastrointestinal hormones; in Johnson LR (ed): Physiology of the Gastrointestinal Tract, ed 3. New York, Raven Press, 1994, pp 1–30.

18 Hildebrand P, Ensinck JW, Gyr K, et al: Evidence for hormonal inhibition of exocrine pancreatic function by somatostatin-28 in humans. Gastroenterology 1992;103:240–247.

19 Harris AG: Somatostatin and somatostatin analogues: Pharmacokinetics and pharmacodynamic effects. Gut 1994;35(suppl):1–4.

20 Gyr KE, Meier R: Pharmacodynamic effects of Sandostatin in the gastrointestinal tract. Digestion 1993;54(suppl 1):14–19.

21 Mottet C, Sieber CC, Nauer A, et al: Hemodynamic effects of the somatostatin analog lanreotide in humans: Placebo-controlled, cross-over dose-ranging echo-Doppler study. Hepatology 1998;27:920–925.

22 Flogstad AK, Halse J, Haldorsen T, et al: Sandostatin LAR in acromegalic patients: A dose-range study. J Clin Endocrinol Metab 1995;80:3601–3607.

23 Grass P, Marbach P, Bruns C, Lancranjan I: Sandostatin LAR (microencapsulated octreotide acetate) in acromegaly: Pharmacokinetic and pharmacodynamic relationships. Metabolism 1996;45(suppl 1):27–30.

24 Gillis JC, Noble S, Goa KL: Octreotide long-acting release. A review of its pharmacological properties and therapeutic use in the management of acromegaly. Drugs 1997;53:681–699.

Digestion

Digestion 1999;60(suppl 2):9–14

The Role of Octreotide in the Treatment of Gastroenteropancreatic Endocrine Tumors

Lukas Degen Christoph Beglinger

Division of Gastroenterology, University Hospital, Basel, Switzerland

Key Words
Carcinoid · Endocrine pancreatic tumors · Somatostatin

Abstract
Gastrointestinal-endocrine pancreatic (GEP) tumors are rare, occurring in less than 1% of the population. They are usually divided into functionally active or nonfunctioning tumors. Functionally active tumors produce a variety of substances (mainly peptides or serotonin). The tumors are classified according to the dominant clinical syndrome that they cause. Surgery is the treatment of choice in patients with GEP tumors and it should always be considered, even if total tumor excision cannot be achieved. Reduction in tumor mass (debulking) may improve the patients symptoms. Medical treatment is used in patients with advanced malignant endocrine tumors. The most important compounds to control symptoms in these patients are somatostatin analogues. Natural somatostatin is produced in different molecular forms and has inhibitory effects on a number of functions. The observation of potent inhibitory effects on various hormone-secreting cells led to the use of somatostatin for symptomatic treatment of peptide-secreting tumors. Natural somatostatin is not suitable for long-term clinical application; therefore, synthetic somatostatin analogues were developed with improved pharmacokinetic characteristics. The best characterized analogue, octreotide, has been successfully applied to patients with functioning GEP tumors. Octreotide can dramatically ameliorate the debilitating symptoms of patients suffering from the clinical manifestations of endocrine tumors such as diarrhea and flushing. The success of octreotide therapy is best reflected in terms of its impact on the patient's quality of life as defined by the activity to perform normal daily activities.

Introduction

Gastrointestinal enteropancreatic endocrine (GEP) tumors are rare – the most common type, the carcinoid tumors, occur in 2–20 persons per 1,000,000 of population. The incidence of the carcinoid syndrome is severalfold lower and estimated to be below 0.5 per 100,000 inhabitants; the incidence for endocrine pancreatic tumors is clearly below this figure [1–3]. The classification used in the literature is unfortunately not uniform; it would be most helpful to include the anatomical location and the predominant hormone production to classify these tumors. Neuroendocrine gastrointestinal and endocrine pancreatic tumors present various clinical pictures with the symptoms primarily related to hormone production. The key characteristics of these tumors is given in table 1.

Several extensive reviews on gut neuroendocrine tumors and their medical management have been published in the last 10 years; a selection is given here and the reader is encouraged to delve into these papers for further reading [1, 2, 4–6]. The present chapter is more focused and presents a summary on the role of somatostatin and

KARGER
Fax +41 61 306 12 34
E-Mail karger@karger.ch
www.karger.ch

0012–2823/99/0608–0009$17.50/0

Accessible online at:
http//BioMedNet.com/karger

Prof. Christoph Beglinger
Division of Gastroenterology, University Hospital
CH–4031 Basel (Switzerland)
Tel. +41 61 2652525/ext 181 2102
Fax +41 61 2653847, E-Mail beglinger@tmr.ch

Table 1. Key characteristics of GEP endocrine tumors

GEP endocrine tumors are rare occurring in less than 1% of the population
Diagnosis of GEP tumors is often complicated and in many cases delayed
GEP endocrine tumors are in general small and their growth is characteristically slow
Symptoms are related to hormone production; they often only appear after metastases are present

somatostatin receptors, on the clinical efficacy of somatostatin analogues (focusing on the somatostatin analogue octreotide) in managing GEP endocrine tumors.

The observation of potent inhibitory effects of somatostatin on different hormone-secreting cells led to the application of the peptide (or synthetic analogues of somatostatin with longer half-lives) in the symptomatic treatment of peptide-secreting tumors. The impressive efficacy of somatostatin therapy in hypersecretory disorders was accompanied by intriguing reports of antiproliferative actions of somatostatin in vitro and in vivo. As mentioned before, this chapter reviews the available literature on the role of somatostatin peptides in the treatment of GEP tumors.

The Functional Importance of Somatostatin Receptors Expressed by GEP Tumors

The variable symptom complexes associated with GEP tumors still create unique difficulties related to the treatment of these tumors. Somatostatin analogues, especially octreotide, have been shown to be therapeutically beneficial in reducing most of the symptoms produced by these tumors. The exact mechanism of action of octreotide in these tumors is still not fully understood [7]. The effect could be a direct one on the tumor tissue itself, it could be related to hormone production as somatostatin analogues can suppress hormone secretion, and/or it could be associated with tumor growth [7, 8]. However, as somatostatin has numerous actions in the body, an indirect effect cannot be excluded (inhibiton of growth factors, inhibition of angiogenesis, modulation of immunological activity).

In a large series of GEP tumors, Reubi et al. [9] have investigated the somatostatin receptor status (62 patients with carcinoid tumors, 15 patients with islet cell carcinomas). These data revealed (a) a high prevalence of somatostatin receptors (at the time of the investigation, the different receptor subtypes were not yet known) in the primary tumors of both carcinoids and islet cell carcinoma; (b) a high prevalence of somatostatin receptors in metastases; (c) a continuous expression of somatostatin receptors during long-term therapy with octreotide; (d) a correlation between the receptor status and the in vivo biochemical response to octreotide treatment. This important paper provides a first rationale basis for treatment strategies and suggests that tumoral somatostatin receptors are the likely molecular basis for octreotide action; the receptors may be an important parameter for predicting the therapeutic efficacy of somatostatin analogues in these tumors. In more recent studies [10–13], somatostatin receptor subtype gene expression was studied in GEP tumors. SSTR2, SSTR4 and SSTR5 messenger RNA transcripts were detected in most cases (92, 82 and 84%, respectively) with SSTR1 and SSTR3 less frequently documented [13]. These data were confirmed by other authors. In one study, in vitro SSTR2 and SSTR5 expression documented a good correlation with in vivo scintigraphy [14]. Octreotide or similar analogues are used as ligands for scintigraphy and these peptides bind with high affinity only to SSTR2 and SSTR5, supporting therefore the hypothesis that the expression of these two receptor subtypes form the molecular basis for the action of octreotide in vivo.

Value of Somatostatin Receptor Scintigraphy for Tumor Localization

Peptide receptor scintigraphy with the radiolabeled somatostatin analogue [^{111}In-DTPA-*D*-Phe]octreotide has become a standard procedure for localizing GEP tumors. Numerous studies [14–17] have documented the ability of this imaging procedure to localize neuroendocrine tumors (carcinoids and islet cell tumors). Most studies have investigated the sensitivity of the modality, but one study has also examined whether somatostatin receptor scintigraphy alters the clinical management of these patients. To achieve a high sensitivity, it is important that SPECT imaging is performed; this capability exists in most nuclear medicine departments. The specificity of the technique is also high. 90–100% of carcinoid tumors, gastrinomas and other pancreatic endocrine tumors possess somatostatin receptors and can be imaged by scintig-

Table 2. The most common GEP tumors and their symptoms

Carcinoid	Most common primary endocrine tumor of the GEP system
	Syndrome characterized by diarrhea, flush and hypertension with increased metabolism of serotonin
Gastrinoma	First described as Zollinger-Ellison syndrome
	Gastrin-producing tumor leading to severe peptic ulcer disease
VIPoma	VIP-producing tumor responsible for watery diarrhea syndrome (endocrine cholera)
Insulinoma	Insulin-producing tumor leading to severe hypoglycemia
Glucagonoma	Excess production of glucagon leading to diabetes and dermatosis (necrolytic migratory rash)

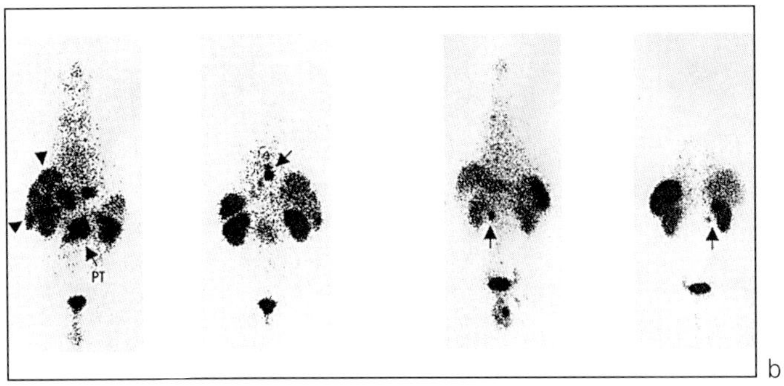

Fig. 1. a,b [^{111}In-DTPA-*D*-Phe]octreotide scintigraphy to localize metastases in a patient with a carcinoid syndrome (courtesy of Prof. H. Bihl, Stuttgart, Germany).

Table 3. Principal aims of octreotide therapy

1.	Improvement of symptoms (hormone suppression)
2.	Inhibition of tumor growth
3.	Improvement in patient's quality of life

raphy; insulinomas are the exception because only 70% have somatostatin receptors [17]. Therefore, based on the available evidence, scintigraphy is an important imaging modality in patients with GEP tumors (examples are given in figure 1a, 1b). It allows imaging of all body areas with high sensitivity and specificity, and has equal or greater sensitivity to other imaging procedures. It should therefore be the initial imaging study of choice in patients with GEP tumors except insulinomas. Its initial use will result in more information that will allow proper management and less expense and inconvenience to the patient.

Treatment Strategies for GEP Endocrine Tumors

It is important to emphasize that patients with GEP endocrine tumors not only die from tumor progression but also from symptoms related to hormone overproduction [1]. The most common tumors and their predominant symptoms are summarized in table 2. Any treatment modality for these patients must include the possibility of surgery. Surgery is still the only treatment that can cure patients with GEP tumors. The goal of surgical procedures is therefore to accurately stage, localize and remove all tumor tissue. Especially in pancreatic endocrine tumors, notably islet cell tumors, the surgeon must realize that some tumors are small and difficult to find. Surgery is still the treatment of choice for local disease or local and regional metastases. If radical, curative surgery cannot be performed, debulking procedures leading to 'tumor mass' reduction must be considered [1, 2, 18, 19]. Only in an advanced disease state, often with multiple liver metastases, other treatment modalities have to be considered. The aims of the medical treatment are threefold: (1) improve symptoms (mainly by suppressing hormone production; (2) reduce tumor growth, and (3) improve the quality of life of these patients (table 3).

Tumor growth varies from one patient to another with some tumors and their metastases remaining unchanged for months or years, while other tumors show explosive growth [8]. In general, however, GEP endocrine tumors grow rather slowly. Aggressive antiproliferative therapy, aside from surgery, include embolization procedures and chemotherapy [1]. Treatment with conventional chemotherapy has been extremely disappointing, while embolization is only possible in selected cases. The introduction of somatostatin analogues for symptomatic treatment of GEP tumors was therefore a major improvement for the management of these patients. The compounds have become the most popular drugs for these indications. Several analogues have become clinically available (octreotide, lanreotide, vapreotide); they all predominantly bind to receptor subtype 2 (SSTR2) and, to a lesser extent, to subtype 5 (SSTR5). The largest database available for information has been obtained with octreotide. Octreotide treatment produces subjective symptomatic improvement in over 70% of patients at doses ranging from 150 to 300 μg/day given usually as three daily subcutaneous injections, but doses up to 1,500 μg/day have been given. The biochemical response, most often expressed as inhibi-

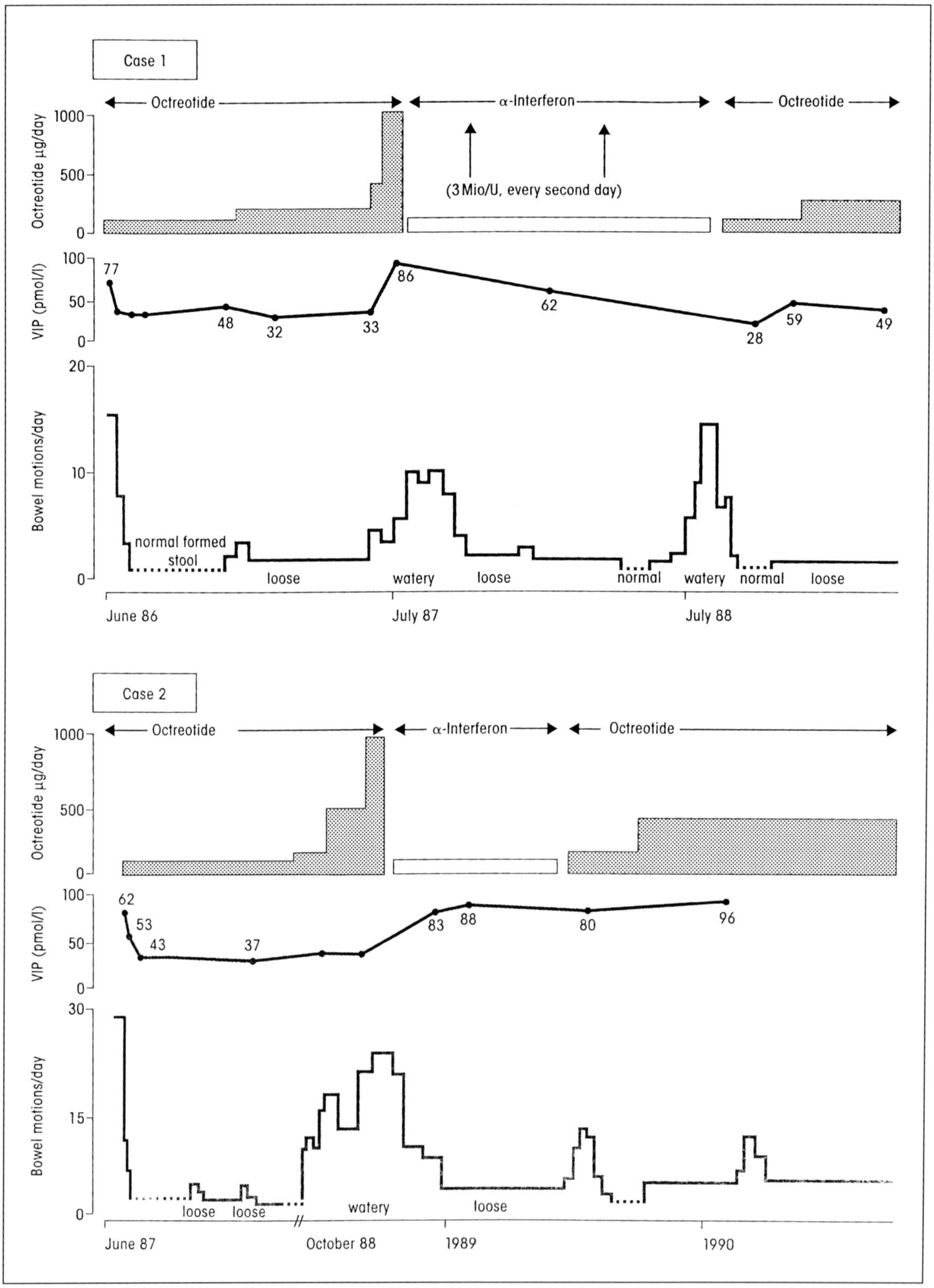

Fig. 2. Illustration of the course of 2 patients with metastatic VIPoma. Typical examples of symptomatic medical treatment of GEP tumors. Both patients were initially treated with octreotide producing a dramatic reduction in daily stool output. In parallel, there was a significant reduction in plasma VIP concentrations (though VIP levels remained above normal values). The treatment was effective for several months in both patients. Thereafter the inhibitory effects of octreotide disappeared and dramatic diarrhea developed again (5–16 liters of stool per day). Both patients were

tion of hormone production, is a little less than symptomatic improvement and the response ranges from 30 to 70% at the same doses [1, 2, 4, 6, 18–20]. Inhibition of tumor growth with octreotide treatment seems to be a rather rare event, but it has been documented in one of the largest clinical trials in patients with metastasized endocrine GEP tumors [21]. The antiproliferative effect can be, at least in selected patients, long-lasting. It has been, however, extremely difficult to demonstrate tumor growth inhibition due to the variable growth kinetics exhibited by these tumors. The therapy with octreotide is well tolerated with only a limited number of well-defined side effects: these include local irritation at the injection site (pain, erythema, swelling), but also abdominal symptoms in the form of pain (cramps, colics) and as steatorrhea as well as mild forms of hyperglycemia. The long-term adverse events are related to the risk of gallstone development; also gallbladder motility is clearly reduced with octreotide treatment, the risk for developing symptomatic gallstone disease with octreotide treatment is only about 1% [5, 22, 23].

The octreotide long-acting release (LAR) formulation, designed for once-monthly intramuscular injection, offers additional quality of life to these patients as the daily subcutaneous injections can be replaced by a single intramuscular injection per month [24–26]. Overall, octreotide LAR has a similar efficacy profile as the subcutaneous formulation and it seems to be well tolerated. The efficacy of octreotide LAR together with a good tolerability profile should enhance patient compliance and contribute to an improvement in patient quality of life. It opens at the same time new therapeutic options. Whether treatment with somatostatin analogues should be combined with α-interferon treatment is still a matter of debate; with octreotide LAR this option can be investigated without extraordinary inconvenience to the patient. α-Interferon was first used as a treatment strategy for advanced GEP endocrine tumors by Oberg and Eriksson [27]. The initial results have been largely confirmed by others [28–30]; the usual doses range from 3 to 9 million units of α-interferon given as subcutaneous injections 3–7 times a week. The efficacy of the initial studies document a symptomatic and biochemical response in up to 50% of patients; in addition, α-interferon should exert antiproliferative effects. The side effects of α-interferon are, however, much higher than those of octreotide. The side effects are clearly dose-dependent and include chronic fatigue, depression, slight anemia and increased liver enzymes. The tolerability profile is therefore unfavorable in comparison to somatostatin analogue treatment. Of interest is the observation that the tolerability of α-interferon is improved when the compound is combined with somatostatin therapy. Based on this information, several randomized, controlled combination trials are ongoing whereby α-interferon is combined with somatostatin analogues. As α-interferon is better tolerated by the patients when combined with somatostatin analogues, a combination of these two compounds could potentially improve efficacy of therapy which could eventually translate into prolonged survival and, more importantly, improve the quality of life of patients with GEP endocrine tumors.

Conclusions

GEP endocrine tumors are rare, occurring in less than 1% of the population. GEP tumors are in general small and their growth is characteristically slow, although some tumors exhibit explosive growth kinetics. Surgery is the primary treatment in patients with GEP tumors and it should always be considered even if total excision cannot be achieved. Reduction in tumor mass (debulking) may improve the patient's symptoms. Most symptoms of advanced disease are related to excessive hormone production. The aim of medical management is therefore to suppress hormone production, which in many cases leads to symptom control. The observation of potent inhibitory effects of somatostatin analogues on various hormone-secreting cells has led to the use of these compounds in peptide-secreting tumors. One of these analogues, octreotide, is available in form of a subcutaneous injection or in form of an intramuscular injection (octreotide LAR). The compound dramatically ameliorates the debilitating symptoms from the clinical manifestations of endocrine tumors such as diarrhea and flushing. The success of octreotide therapy is reflected in terms of its impact on the patient's quality of life as defined by the ability to perform normal daily activities.

changed to treatment with α-interferon which induced remission of diarrhea. The α-interferon treatment was effective for a few moths, then profuse watery diarrhea occurred again and the patients were successfully started on a second course of octreotide. Loss of control of symptoms occurred with both octreotide and α-interferon treatment. A cross-over in the treatment can induce dramatic responses. Recent observations suggest combined administration of octreotide (preferably as octreotide LAR) and α-interferon.

References

1 Oberg K: Neuroendocrine gastrointestinal tumours. Ann Oncol 1996;7:453–463.
2 Arnold R, Frank M: Gastrointestinal endocrine tumours: Medical management. Baillières Clin Gastroenterol 1996;10:737–759.
3 Bloom SR, Polak JM: Somatostatin. Br Med J 1987;295:288–290.
4 Bajetta E, Carnaghi C, Ferrari L, Spagnoli I, Mazzaferro V, Buzzoni R: The role of somatostatin analogues in the treatment of gastroenteropancreatic endocrine tumours. Digestion 1996; 57(suppl 1):72–76.
5 Battershill PE, Clissold SP: Octreotide. A review of its pharmacodynamic and pharmacokinetic properties, and therapeutic potential in conditions associated with excessive peptide secretion. Drugs 1989;38:658–702.
6 Oberg K, Norheim I, Theodorsson E: Treatment of malignant midgut carcinoid tumours with a long-acting somatostatin analogue octreotide. Acta Oncol 1991;30:503–507.
7 Yamada T, Creutzfeldt W, Beglinger C, Chiba T: The effect of somatostatin on cellular proliferation. Gastroenterol Int 1994;7:13–23.
8 Arnold R, Frank M: Control of growth in neuroendocrine gastro-enteropancreatic tumours. Digestion 1996;57(suppl 1):69–71.
9 Reubi JC, Kvols LK, Waser B, et al: Detection of somatostatin receptors in surgical and percutaneous needle biopsy samples of carcinoids and islet cell carcinomas. Cancer Res 1990;50:5969–5977.
10 Viollet C, Prevost G, Maubert E, et al: Molecular pharmacology of somatostatin receptors. Fundam Clin Pharmacol 1995;9:107–113.
11 Panetta R, Patel YC: Expression of mRNA for all five human somatostatin receptors (hSSTR1-5) in pituitary tumors. Life Sci 1995;56:333–342.
12 Epelbaum J, Bertherat J, Prevost G, et al: Molecular and pharmacological characterization of somatostatin receptor subtypes in adrenal, extraadrenal, and malignant pheochromocytomas. J Clin Endocrinol Metab 1995;80:1837–1844.
13 Jais P, Terris B, Ruszniewski P, et al: Somatostatin receptor subtype gene expression in human endocrine gastroentero-pancreatic tumours. Eur J Clin Invest 1997;27:639–644.
14 John M, Meyerhof W, Richter D, et al: Positive somatostatin receptor scintigraphy correlates with the presence of somatostatin receptor subtype 2. GUT 1996;38:33–39.
15 Krenning EP, Bakker WH, Breeman WA, et al: Localisation of endocrine-related tumours with radioiodinated analogue of somatostatin. Lancet 1989;i:242–244.
16 Lamberts SW, Bakker WH, Reubi JC, Krenning EP: Somatostatin-receptor imaging in the localization of endocrine tumors. N Engl J Med 1990; 323:1246–1249.
17 Termanini B, Gibril F, Reynolds JC, et al: Value of somatostatin receptor scintigraphy: A prospective study in gastrinoma of its effect on clinical management. Gastroenterology 1997;112: 335–347.
18 Lamberts SW, Reubi JC, Krenning EP: The role of somatostatin analogs in the control of tumor growth. Semin Oncol 1994;21(suppl 13):61–64.
19 Lamberts SW, Krenning EP, Reubi JC: The role of somatostatin and its analogs in the diagnosis and treatment of tumors. Endocr Rev 1991;12: 450–482.
20 di Bartolomeo M, Bajetta E, Buzzoni R, et al: Clinical efficacy of octreotide in the treatment of metastatic neuroendocrine tumors. A study by the Italian Trials in Medical Oncology Group. Cancer 1996;77:402–408.
21 Arnold R, Trautmann ME, Creutzfeldt W, et al: Somatostatin analogue octreotide and inhibition of tumour growth in metastatic endocrine gastroenteropancreatic tumours. Gut 1996;38: 430–438.
22 Harris AG: Somatostatin and somatostatin analogues: Pharmacokinetics and pharmacodynamic effects. Gut 1994;35(suppl):1–4.
23 Trendle MC, Moertel CG, Kvols LK: Incidence and morbidity of cholelithiasis in patients receiving chronic octreotide for metastatic carcinoid and malignant islet cell tumors. Cancer 1997;79:830–834.
24 Stewart PM, Kane KF, Stewart SE, Lancranjan I, Sheppard MC: Depot long-acting somatostatin analog (Sandostatin-LAR) is an effective treatment for acromegaly. J Clin Endocrinol Metab 1995;80:3267–3272.
25 Lancranjan I, Bruns C, Grass P: Sandostatin LAR: Pharmacokinetics, efficacy, and tolerability in acromegalic patients. Metabolism 1995; 44:18–26.
26 Gillis JC, Noble S, Goa KL: Octreotide long-acting release (LAR). A review of its pharmacological properties and therapeutic use in the management of acromegaly. Drugs 1997;53: 681–699.
27 Oberg K, Eriksson B: The role of interferons in the management of carcinoid tumours. Br J Haematol 1991;79(suppl 1):74–77.
28 Oberg K: Interferon-alpha versus somatostatin or the combination of both in gastro-enteropancreatic tumours. Digestion 1996;57(suppl 1): 81–83.
29 Faiss S, Scherubl H, Riecken EO, Wiedenmann B: Interferon-alpha versus somatostatin or the combination of both in metastatic neuroendocrine gut and pancreatic tumours. Digestion 1996;57(suppl 1):84–85.
30 Creutzfeldt W, Bartsch HH, Jacubaschke U, Stockmann F: Treatment of gastrointestinal endocrine tumours with interferon-alpha and octreotide. Acta Oncol 1991;30:529–535.

Digestion

Digestion 1999;60(suppl 2):15–22

The Role of Octreotide in the Prevention of Complications following Pancreatic Resection

Pascal O. Berberat Helmut Friess Waldemar Uhl Markus W. Büchler

Department of Visceral and Transplantation Surgery, University of Bern, Inselspital, Bern, Switzerland

Key Words

Octreotide · Pancreas · Pancreatic carcinoma · Chronic pancreatitis · Surgery

Abstract

Postoperative complications following major pancreatic surgery are mainly due to the difficulties of performing a safe and proper anastomosis between the stomach or small bowel and the pancreas. Continuous pancreatic juice secretion and the often soft structure of the pancreatic parenchyma are major risk factors.

The present paper summarizes the results of six previously published, placebo-controlled, double-blind trials and one open randomized trial analyzing the efficacy of octreotide in preventing postoperative complications in patients who undergo major pancreatic surgery. Patients were given either octreotide (3 × 100–150 μg subcutaneously/day) or a placebo perioperatively for 5–7 days starting at least 1 h before operation. The patients were monitored postoperatively for typical postoperative complications such as: leakage of the anastomosis, pancreatic fistula, abscess, fluid collection, shock, sepsis, pulmonary insufficiency, renal insufficiency, bleeding, postoperative pancreatitis, and death.

Six of the seven studies showed significantly fewer postoperative complications in the octreotide group in comparison with the placebo group ($p < 0.05$). The effectiveness of octreotide was most apparent in the prevention of secretion-related complications such as fistula, fluid collection and leakage of the anastomosis.

These studies demonstrated that inhibition of perioperative pancreatic secretion is a viable treatment concept in patients undergoing major pancreatic surgery. The perioperative and prophylactic application of octreotide in patients who undergo major pancreatic resection reduces the postoperative complication rate significantly.

Introduction

Although mortality rates following major pancreatic surgery have decreased continuously in recent years, they still average 10%, and medical and surgical postoperative complications occur in approximately 40% of patients who undergo major pancreatic surgery [1–5].

Postoperative complications such as insufficiency of the pancreaticojejunal anastomosis, pancreatic fistula, peripancreatic fluid collection and abscess are chiefly associated with two risk factors: (1) the technical difficulties of performing a proper and safe anastomosis between the pancreatic remnant and the intestine (stomach, jejunum), and (2) exocrine pancreatic secretion, which might cause tension on the pancreaticointestinal anastomosis.

Both risk factors are closely associated with the texture of the remaining pancreas, because a critical aspect of suturing the intestinopancreatic anastomosis is the consistency of the pancreatic parenchyma [3, 6, 7]. A recent review of the literature including 2,664 patients with Whipple resection underlines the importance of the pancreatic texture with regard to postoperative complications

KARGER

Fax + 41 61 306 12 34
E-Mail karger@karger.ch
www.karger.ch

0012–2823/99/0608–0015$17.50/0

Accessible online at:
http//BioMedNet.com/karger

Markus W. Büchler, MD
Department of Visceral and Transplantation Surgery
University of Bern, Inselspital
CH–3010 Bern (Switzerland)
Tel. +41 31 632 24 04, Fax +41 31 382 47 72, E-Mail markus.buechler@insel.ch

[3]. This review found a postoperative fistula rate of 5% in chronic pancreatitis, 12% in pancreatic cancer, 15% in ampullary cancer and 33% in bile duct cancer. The mortality rate in patients with a fistula was 9% in chronic pancreatitis, 31% in pancreatic cancer, 27% in periampullary cancer and 70% in bile duct cancers. These findings support the hypothesis that postoperative complications following major pancreatic surgery are closely related to the morphology of the pancreatic remnant. Similar conclusions were reached in a recent analysis in which postoperative complications were compared with the size and the degree of fibrosis of the remnant gland. In 74 patients there was a clear relationship between postoperative complications and the secretion capacity of the remaining pancreas [7].

Postoperative complications following pancreatic resection are often caused by pancreatic juice that leaks from the pancreatic remnant and reaches the peripancreatic region or even the free abdominal cavity. The subsequent actions of activated proteases such as elastase or trypsin can cause severe inflammation and may lead to the autodestruction of peripancreatic tissues. The sometimes fatal outcome after leakage of the pancreatic anastomosis with sudden life-threatening hemorrhage is explained by this sequence of events [8, 9].

Based on this hypothesis, inhibition of exocrine pancreatic secretion should improve the postoperative course and consequently reduce postoperative complications after pancreatic resection.

The concept of inhibiting exocrine pancreatic secretion to prevent postoperative complications originated in 1979 [10]. In a small, uncontrolled trial, a continuous intravenous infusion (250 μg/h) of somatostatin-14 was administered perioperatively to patients undergoing Whipple's resection. The authors reported a reduction in the postoperative complication rate, including a lower occurrence of postoperative acute pancreatitis. The human hormone somatostatin has been demonstrated to strongly inhibit basal and stimulated exocrine pancreatic secretion [11, 12]. The synthetic somatostatin analogue octreotide is known as a potent inhibitor of exocrine pancreatic secretion. Due to its longer serum and biological half-life, it is more convenient than native somatostatin for clinical use [13, 14].

The value of perioperative administration of octreotide has been investigated in five randomized, placebo-controlled, double-blind, multicentric trials which were performed in Germany, Italy and France. Additionally, two smaller, single-institution prospective randomized trials were performed in Spain and in the USA [15–21].

In the present paper we summarize the results of these seven studies. The first multicenter octreotide trial in major pancreatic surgery was carried out in Germany between 1989 and 1990 [15]. The patients were stratified into a high-risk group and a low-risk group. Patients undergoing pancreatic operation due to benign or malignant pancreatic or peripancreatic tumors (soft pancreas) were assigned to the high-risk group, whereas patients with chronic pancreatitis (firm pancreas) were assigned to the low-risk group. The second German octreotide multicenter study was designed based on the results of the first German trial, but enrolled only patients with chronic pancreatitis [17]. In a trial similar to the first German octreotide study, the first Italian octreotide study group stratified its patients into a high-risk (tumor) patient group and a low-risk (chronic pancreatitis) group [16]. The second Italian octreotide study summarized all patients [18]. A single-institution trial was performed in Spain [19]. Recently, an additional single-institution trial, performed in the USA, enrolled only patients with malignant disease [20]. Finally, in 1998 another prospective, placebo-controlled, double-blind, multicentric trial was presented by a French group [21]. However, this study is presently only available as an abstract and therefore the data cannot be reported in full detail.

Study Design of Multicentric Octreotide Studies in Pancreatic Surgery

The study protocols used in the two German and the two Italian multicentric octreotide trials were similar and were based on the protocol which was originally used in the first German octreotide study [14]. Patients suffering from a pancreatic tumor or chronic pancreatitis who were suitable for pancreatic resection or pancreatic duct anastomosis were enrolled in the study after giving written, informed consent. On the day before the operation, the patients who satisfied the inclusion criteria were randomly assigned to receive a 7-day treatment of either 3×100 μg octreotide (1 ml volume; Sandoz AG, Nürnberg, Germany; Sandoz Prodotti Farmaceutici, Milan, Italy) subcutaneously (every 8 h) or 21 subcutaneous placebo injections (1 ml each) in a double-blinded manner. Each patient treatment was initiated at least 1 h before laparotomy. The octreotide dosage of 3×100 μg subcutaneously/day was chosen after a pilot trial had shown that this dosage maximally inhibits exocrine pancreatic secretion in humans [18–20]. Each patient received intravenous antibiotic prophylaxis perioperatively for 24–48 h with antibacterial drugs effective against intestinal germs. Postoperatively, the patients were treated in an intensive care unit. Intravenous crystalloid solutions were administered (2.5–3 liters/day) according to clinical requirements, and these were supplemented by plasma or blood components in order to maintain a positive central venous pressure and a blood hematocrit ≥30%. The patients were permitted nothing orally for at least the first 3 postoperative days. Each patient was followed up until the 90th postoperative day. The study protocols were approved by the ethics committees of each participating hospital and were in compliance with the clinical practice guidelines of the European Community.

Definition of Postoperative Complications

Eleven typical postoperative complications following pancreatic resection were defined, and the patients were monitored in a standardized manner to detect them [14, 16].

Death	within 90 days postoperatively.
Leakage	from pancreatic, biliary, or intestinal anastomosis as determined by radiographic or intraoperative findings (relaparotomy).
Pancreatic fistula	if (1) the concentrations of amylase and lipase in the drainage fluid were >3 times higher than in the serum of n consecutive postoperative days and (2) a drainage volume of >10 ml/24 h was present, a pancreatic fistula was defined. The serum and drainage fluid amylase and/or lipase concentrations were determined on postoperative days 1, 3, 4, 5 and 7 and twice weekly thereafter.
Intra-abdominal abscess	was defined as pus collection or infected fluid collection revealed by either ultrasound or computed tomography (CT)-guided needle aspiration and microbiological culture or demonstrated at time of relaparotomy.
Intra-abdominal fluid collection	(sterile) was defined as a collection of fluid at least 5 cm in diameter which was identified by ultrasound or CT but which did not qualify as an abscess. All patients were screened for a fluid collection by means of ultrasound or CT on days 4 and 8 postoperatively.
Cardiocirculatory shock	was defined as a systolic blood pressure of <80 mm Hg for more than 20 min at some point (later than 24 h postoperatively) which required continuous volume replacement and/or treatment with catecholamines.
Sepsis	was defined as the presence of at least four of the following criteria: (1) bacterial-positive blood culture; (2) rectal temperature >38.5 °C; (3) leukocytosis >12,000/mm^3 or leukopenia <3,000/mm^3; (4) thrombocytopenia <100,000/mm^3, and (5) metabolic acidosis (base excess > −4). Blood cultures were taken daily in patients with rectal temperature >38.5 °C. Blood leukocyte and thrombocyte determination and blood gas analysis were performed on postoperative days 1, 3, 4, 5 and 7 and twice weekly afterwards.
Pulmonary insufficiency	was defined as an arterial pO_2 of <60 mm Hg, despite oxygen application (4 liters/min) via the nose, or when the patient required prolonged postoperative mechanical ventilation (for >24 h after the end of surgery) or reintubation.
Renal insufficiency	was defined as an increase in serum creatinine of more than twice the preoperative value. Patients whose serum creatinine was increased preoperatively (>120 mmol/l) were not included in the analysis of this criterion. Serum creatinine was monitored on postoperative days 1, 3, 4, 5 and 7 and twice weekly afterwards.
Bleeding	was defined as the replacement of >3 units of blood at least 24 h after the end of surgery or the indication for relaparotomy due to intra-abdominal or intra-intestinal bleeding. Hematocrit was monitored daily on postoperative days 1, 3, 4, 5 and 7 and twice weekly afterwards.
Postoperative acute pancreatitis	was defined as a more than threefold increase in serum amylase or lipase on postoperative day 4 or later, accompanied by morphological signs of acute pancreatitis by contrast-enhanced CT scan. CT was mandatory in patients with a threefold increase in serum amylase or lipase on postoperative days 4 or later.

Results

First German Multicenter Study on Octreotide in Pancreatic Surgery (*Carcinoma and Chronic Pancreatitis*) [15]

The first German multicentric trial was carried out between October 1989 and July 1990 in 18 centers for pancreatic surgery. The study protocol stratified patients into two risk groups: (a) patients with pancreatic or periampullary tumors (soft pancreas) and (b) patients with chronic pancreatitis (firm pancreas), in whom the postoperative complication rate is normally lower than in tumors.

In total, 246 patients with pancreatic or periampullary tumors or severe chronic pancreatitis undergoing surgery were suitable for final evaluation in this prospective investigation. 125 patients were assigned to the octreotide group and 121 to the placebo group. The octreotide group and the placebo group were homogeneous for age, gender, type of operation, and underlying disease. The majority of patients underwent either a partial pancreaticoduodenectomy (Whipple's operation, 61.8%) or a duodenoum-preserving pancreatic head resection (19.5%); the other patients underwent a pancreatic left resection (12.6%), a pancreaticojejunostomy (3.3%), an enucleation (1.2%), or another operative technique (1.6%).

Mortality within 90 days following surgery was 4.5% (11/246 patients, 4 patients from the octreotide and 7 patients from the placebo group). 40 patients (32%) in the octreotide group and 67 patients (55.4%) in the placebo group suffered from one or more postoperative complications. This difference was significant at a level of $p<0.005$. The most frequent complication was pancreatic fistula (27.6%), followed by pulmonary insufficiency (11.4%), bleeding and abscess (8.9 and 8.1%, respectively), fluid collection (6.9%), leakage of the anastomosis (5.3%), shock (5.3%), sepsis (3.7%), postoperative pancreatitis (1.6%) and renal insufficiency (1.2%). The frequency of death, pancreatic fistula, abscess, sepsis, pulmonary insufficiency, and postoperative pancreatitis was lower in the octreotide group than in the placebo group. Postoperatively, serum pancreatic enzymes were lower in the patients receiving octreotide.

When the patients were stratified in the high-risk group (tumors) and in the low-risk group (chronic pancreatitis) the rates of complications among the high-risk patients were 38% for the octreotide group and 65% for the placebo group ($p<0.01$). A similar trend was found in the low-risk group; however, the difference in complication rates between octreotide (25%) and placebo (42%) was not statistically significant ($p=0.057$).

The study medication was well tolerated by most patients. 33 patients with octreotide treatment (26.4%) and 28 patients with placebo treatment (23.1%) exhibited minor side effects. These included burning at the injection side (octreotide 31 patients; placebo 25 patients), hot flashes (2 patients in the octreotide group), inflammatory reaction at the injection site (1 patient in the placebo group) and itching (2 patients in the placebo group).

Second German Multicenter Study on Octreotide in Surgery of Chronic Pancreatitis [17]

The second German multicentric octreotide trial was carried out using the same study protocol as in the first trial. 280 patients were recruited in this study but 33 were withdrawn from the final evaluation either because there was an intraoperative diagnosis of pancreatic cancer or because no pancreatic resection had been performed according to the inclusion criteria. Thus 247 patients were evaluated, with 122 subsequently asigned to the octreotide group and 125 to the placebo group. The patients underwent either a Whipple resection (28%), pancreaticojejunostomy (25%), pancreatic left resection (22%), duodenum-preserving pancreatic head resection (22%), or other operative procedures (3%).

The overall mortality rate within 90 days postoperatively was 1.2% (3/247 patients). Two patients (1.6%) in the octreotide group and 1 patient (0.8%) in the placebo group died. The total complication rate was 23.1% (57/247 patients). 20 patients (16.4%) in the octreotide group and 37 patients (29.6%) in the placebo group suffered from one or more complications postoperatively. This difference was significant at a level of $p=0.007$ (Fisher's exact test used for statistical analysis).

No severe side effects of the octreotide therapy could be found. Even the serum glucose levels (median) followed nearly the same course in the octreotide and placebo groups. 59 events (24 octreotide, 35 placebo) were observed which might have been side effects of the study medication. 42 patients (18 octreotide, 24 placebo) experienced some pain, burning or erythema at the injection site but none required discontinuation of the treatment. Eleven other patients (4 octreotide, 7 placebo) suffered from nausea, vomiting, heartburn, diarrhea and intestinal cramps, which likewise did not necessitate discontinuation of the treatment. Two patients (1 octreotide, 1 placebo) suffered from hyperglycemia, which again did not necessitate discontinuation of the treatment. In addition, 1 patient in the octreotide group developed dyspopia and

1 patient in the placebo group had disturbance of coagulation, which disappeared without further therapy and did not necessitate discontinuation of the treatment. No further side effects were recorded in this trial.

First Italian Multicenter Study on Octreotide in Pancreatic Surgery [16]

In the first Italian multicentric trial, 252 patients were included who were suffering from pancreatic or periampullary carcinoma or chronic pancreatitis. The study protocol and the definitions of the monitored postoperative complications were similar to the first German octreotide study. 122 subjects were assigned to the octreotide group and 130 to the placebo group. The majority of the patients underwent a Whipple resection (39.7%), a pancreaticojejunostomy (26.2%) or a left pancreatectomy (23.8%), while the remaining patients underwent enucleation (5.6%), intermediate resection (2.8%) or duodenum-preserving pancreatic head resection (2%). The octreotide group and the placebo group were homogeneous for age, gender, type of operation and underlying disease. Seven patients died within 90 days postoperatively (2.8%): 2 patients in the octreotide group (1.5%) and 5 patients in the placebo group (3.8%).

Nineteen octreotide patients (15.6% of the octreotide group) and 38 placebo patients (29.2% of the placebo group) suffered from one or more complications postoperatively. The total complication rate was 22.6% (57/252 patients). The most frequent complication was pancreatic fistula, in 11 octreotide patients (9% of the octreotide group) versus 24 placebo patients (18.5% of the placebo group), followed by fluid collection (8 octreotide patients (6.6%) versus 13 placebo patients (10%)), sepsis (2 octreotide patients (1.6%) versus 8 placebo patients (6.1%)), anastomotic leakage (4 octreotide patients (3.3%) versus 5 placebo patients (3.8%)), and abscess (3 octreotide patients (2.5%) versus 6 placebo patients (4.6%)).

Moderate to severe side effects were reported in 4 patients, all of whom received octreotide. Febrile rash in 1 patient caused withdrawal of the treatment after 5 days, but the rash subsequently resolved without further therapy. Skin rash developed in 1 patient and vomiting in another, but both episodes were mild and resolved spontaneously. In an additional patient, biliary sludge was observed on routine ultrasonography. No differences were observed between the two groups in the proportion of patients with altered vital signs and laboratory variables. In patients receiving octreotide, no significant changes were observed in blood glucose levels.

Second Italian Multicenter Study on Octreotide in Pancreatic Surgery [18]

In the second Italian multicentric trial, 218 patients suffering from neoplastic or chronic inflammatory diseases of the pancreas and the periampullary region were recruited between July 1990 and May 1992. The vast majority of these patients undergoing pancreatic resection suffered from cancer, with chronic pancreatitis accounting for only 8.2% of patients. 111 patients were assigned to the octreotide group and 107 to the placebo group. The two groups were homogeneous for age, gender, types of operations, and underlying disease. The majority underwent either a Whipple resection (39.9%), a duodenum-preserving pancreatic head resection (25.7%) or a pancreatic left resection (24.8%); the other patients underwent a subtotal pancreatectomy (5.5%), an enucleation (2.3%) or another operation technique (1.8%).

The overall postoperative mortality rate was 6.9% (15/218 patients): 8.1% (9/111 patients) in the octreotide group and 5.6% (6/107 patients) in the placebo group. 63 patients had one or more postoperative complications, which accounts for an overall morbidity rate of 28.9%. Among these, 24 were octreotide patients (21.6% of the octreotide group) and 39 were placebo patients (36.4% of the placebo group), with a statistically significant difference ($p < 0.05$). Pancreatic fistula was the most frequent complication. It occurred in 31 of the 218 patients (14.2%): in 9% of the octreotide and in 19.6% of the placebo group, with a significant difference ($p < 0.05$). Bleeding was reported in 7.8% of the patients, anastomotic leakage in 5.5%, fluid collection in 5%, postoperative pancreatitis in 3.2%, abscess in 3.2%, respiratory failure in 1.8%, renal failure in 0.5% and other complications in 5% of the patients.

Six patients (2.8) showed side effects: 2 nausea, 2 vomiting, 1 diarrhea, 1 prolonged bowel transit; 3 of these patients were in the octreotide and 3 in the placebo group.

Spanish Single-Institution Study on Octreotide in Pancreatic Surgery [19]

This Spanish single-institution, prospective, randomized and placebo-controlled trial included 34 patients who underwent pancreaticoduodenectomy because of benign and malignant pancreatic disease. 16 patients were assigned to receive octreotide and 18 patients were treated with a placebo.

Overall postoperative mortality was 3% and morbidity was 26%. There were no differences in the total number of complications between the octreotide and placebo groups, but there was a significantly smaller number of pancreatic fistulas in the octreotide group (0 vs. 5, $p=0.03$). There was no statistical difference in the occurrence of pancreatic fistula in relation to the nature of the disease (3 in the normal and 2 in the fibrotic pancreas). In addition, the number of relaparotomies and the length of the postoperative hospital stay were significantly shorter in the octreotide group compared with the placebo group ($p<0.05$).

American Single-Institution Study on Octreotide in Pancreatic Surgery (Only Carcinoma) [20]

In this American single-institution, prospective, open, randomized trial, 110 patients were enrolled between June 1991 and December 1995. The study included only patients who underwent a pancreaticoduodenectomy for malignancy. At the time of surgery the patients were randomized to receive 150 μg octreotide 3 times a day for 5 days or nothing. The first dose of octreotide was given in the operating room after surgery was finished or when the patient arrived in the intensive care unit. The two groups were homogeneous for demographics, treatment variables and histological diagnosis. 17 patients (30%) in the octreotide group and 13 patients (25%) in the control group suffered from one or more postoperative complications. This difference was not statistically significant.

The most frequent complication was pancreatic fistula (49% total, 18% clinical). The incidence of clinical pancreatic anastomotic leak was 12% (7/57) in the octreotide group and 6% (3/53) in the control group. There were no significant differences with regard to reoperations and length of hospital stay between the two groups.

French Multicenter Study on Octreotide in Pancreatic Surgery [21]

In this multicenter, prospective, randomized, double-blind and placebo-controlled trial conducted by a French surgical group, 230 patients were included. There was a significant difference in the postoperative complication rate between the octreotide group and the placebo group following both the Whipple resection (17 vs. 45%) and pancreaticojejunostomy (24 vs. 41%).

Discussion

Somatostatin, a tetradecapeptide originally discovered in hypothalamic tissue, is a powerful inhibitor of basal and stimulated exocrine pancreatic secretion [11, 12]. Its action on the pancreas is mediated via the inhibition of secretagogue gastrointestinal hormones and by direct pathways via somatostatin receptors on acinar cells [25]. Octreotide (SMS 201-995), an octapeptide analogue of somatostatin, was synthesized to have more specific, more potent and longer-acting inhibitory effects than native somatostatin [13, 14, 26]. In particular, the longer half-life of octreotide (100 min) in comparison with somatostatin-14 (2–3 min) has made this compound preferable for clinical application. Octreotide can be given 3 times daily due to its biological action of 8–10 h. In a pilot trial, we were able to show that 100 μg octreotide, administered subcutaneously, inhibited the stimulated secretion of amylase, trypsin, and chymotrypsin by 84, 76 and 77%, respectively [22–24]. Our data confirmed those of earlier reports which showed a maximum inhibition of pancreatic protease and amylase secretion with comparable dosages of octreotide.

In pancreatic resection, the anastomosis of the pancreatic remnant to the stomach or small bowel constitutes the major risk factor [3, 6]. This problem is mainly technical, given the difficulties associated with performing a proper and safe anastomosis with this often smooth organ [6]. Typical postoperative complications are linked with exocrine pancreatic secretion from the pancreatic remnant (including harmful proteases and lipolytic enzymes) and the friability of the anastomosis.

The concept of perioperative inhibition of exocrine pancreatic secretion by intravenous somatostatin infusion dates back to 1979. In an open trial, Klempa et al. [10] were able to show a drop in postoperative morbidity including reduced occurrence of acute pancreatitis following Whipple's resection. Two other groups have used the somatostatin analogue octreotide to prevent pancreatic fistula and acute pancreatitis following pancreatic transplantation [27, 28].

The ability of octreotide to prevent complications in patients undergoing major pancreatic surgery has been investigated in two multicentric, placebo-controlled, double-blinded studies carried out in Germany by our group [15, 17], in two studies carried out in Italy [16, 18] and in one French study [21] using a comparable study design. Recently, two additional prospective, randomized trials have addressed this topic: a small single-institution trial in Spain and one in the USA. In all five multicenter studies and the small Spanish single-institution trial, the postoperative complication rate was significantly lower in patients with octreotide treatment than in patients who received a placebo. Only in the American single-institution trial was there no difference in the postoperative complication rate found between patients receiving octreotide and a placebo.

It should be noted that, besides the fact that the American study was not double-blinded and placebo-controlled, octreotide was not given prophylactically. Whereas in the multicentric studies octreotide was given before the operation, in the USA study it was delayed until either the reconstruction was finished or the whole operation was done. The idea with octreotide is to inhibit pancreatic secretion and thereby to remove tension from the pancreatic anastomosis. In this way the pancreatic anastomosis can heal faster and thereby postoperative complications can be lowered. To achieve this effect, octreotide has to be given before the anastomosis is performed. Also, the postoperative observation time in the American trial was only 30 days, whereas in the other studies the patients were followed until the 90th postoperative day. Also of possible importance is the fact that only pancreatic cancer patients were included. This means that – based on their soft pancreatic tissue – all patients would have been assigned to the high-risk group for postoperative complications. However, in patients who received preoperative chemoradiation, the pancreas could have shown a more firm texture (fibrosis), with subsequently decreased pancreatic exocrine function. Therefore, most of the patients in this study would actually belong in the low-risk group according to the definition in the first German octreotide trial, and a much higher number of patients is required to prove the efficacy of octreotide in preventing postoperative complications.

The main disadvantage of the American study is its open design (not double-blind). As we know from our own experience and from a number of scientific investigations, the bias of an investigator is of major influence in the outcome of these studies.

In summary, the overall results in the prophylactic perioperative application of the somatostatin analogue octreotide at a daily dosage of 3×100 μg subcutaneously in patients undergoing elective pancreatic surgery for pancreatic or periampullary carcinoma or chronic pancreatitis indicate that the occurrence of typical postoperative complications can be significantly reduced.

References

1 Jordan GL Jr: Pancreatic resection for pancreatic cancer; in Howard JM, Jordan GL Jr, Reber HA (eds): Surgical Diseases of the Pancreas. Philadelphia, Lea & Febiger, 1987, pp 666–714.

2 Howard JM: Surgical treatment of chronic pancreatitis; in Howard JM, Jordan GL Jr, Reber HA (eds): Surgical Diseases of the Pancreas. Philadelphia, Lea & Febiger 1987, pp 496–521.

3 Bartoli FG, Arnone GB, Ravera G, Bach V: Pancreatic fistulas and relative mortality in malignant disease after pancreaticoduodenectomy. Review and statistical meta-analysis regarding 15 years of literature. Anticancer Res 1991;11:1831–1848.

4 Friess H, Müller MW, Büchler MW: Duodenum-preserving pancreatic head resection: The future. Dig Surg 1994;11:318–324.

5 Bramhall SR, Allum WH, Jones AG, Allwood A, Cummins C, Neoptolemos JP: Treatment and survival in 13,560 patients with pancreatic cancer, and incidence of the disease, in the West Midlands: An epidemiological study. Br J Surg 1995;82:111–115.

6 Friess H, Malfertheiner P, Isenmann R, Kühne H, Beger HG, Büchler MW: The risk of the pancreatico-intestinal anastomosis can be predicted preoperatively. Pancreas 1996;13:202–208.

7 Al Sharaf Ch, Ishe I, Dawiskiba S, Andrén-Sandberg A: Characteristics of the gland remnant predict complications after subtotal pancreatectomy. Dig. Surg 1997;14:101–106.

8 Pellegrini CA, Heck CF, Raper S, Way LW: An analysis of the reduced morbidity and mortality rates after pancreaticoduodenectomy. Arch Surg 1989;124:778–781.

9 Trede M, Schwall G: The complications of pancreatectomy. Ann Surg 1988;207:39–47.

10 Klempa J, Schwedes U, Usadel KH: Verhütung von postoperativen pankreatischen Komplikationen nach Duodenopankreatektomie durch Somatostatin. Chirurg 1979;50:427–432.

11 Raptis S, Schlegel W, Lehmann E, Dollinger HC, Zoupas Ch: Effects of somatostatin on the exocrine pancreas and the release of duodenal hormones. Metabolism 1978;27:1321–1328.

12 Creutzfeldt W, Lankisch PG, Fölsch UR: Hemmung der Secretin- und Cholecystokinin-Pancreozymin-induzierten Saft- und Enzymsekretion des Pankreas und der Gallenblasenkontraktion bei Menschen durch Somatostatin. Dtsch Med Wochenschr 1975;100:1135–1138.

13 Köhler E, Beglinger Ch, Dettwiler S, Whitehouse I, Gyr K: Effect of a new somatostatin analogue on pancreatic function in healthy volunteers. Pancreas 1986;2:154–159.

14 Lembcke B, Creutzfeldt W, Schleser S, Ebert R, Shaw C, Koop I: Effect of the somatostatin analogue sandostatin (SMS 201-995) on gastrointestinal, pancreatic and biliary function and hormone release in normal men. Digestion 1987;36:108–124.

15 Büchler M, Friess H, Klempa I, Hermanek P, Sulkowski U, Becker H, Schafmayer A, Baca I, Lorenz D, Meister R, Kremar B, Wagner P, Witte J, Zurmayer EL, Saeger HD, Rieck B, Dollinger P, Glaser K, Teichmann R, Konradt J, Gans W, Dennler HJ, Walzel P, Beger HG: Role of octreotide in the prevention of postoperative complications following pancreatic resection. Am J Surg 1992;163:125–130.

16 Pederzoli P, Bassi C, Falconi M, Camboni M: Efficacy of octreotide in the prevention of complications of elective pancreatic surgery. Br J Surg 1994;81:265–269.

17 Friess H, Beger HG, Sulkowski U, Becker H, Hofbauer B, Dennler HJ, Büchler MW: Randomized controlled milticentre study of the prevention of complications by octreotide in patients undergoing surgery for chronic pancreatitis. Br J Surg 1995;82:1270–1273.

18 Montorsi M, Zago M, Mosca F, Capussotti L, Zotti E, Ribotta G, Fegiz G, Fissi S, Roviaro G, Peracchia A, Pivi M, Perego R, Pezzuoli G: Efficacy of octreotide in the prevention of pancreatic fistula after elective pancreatic resections: A prospective, controlled, randomized clinical trial. Surgery 1995;117:26–31.

19 Briceno Delgado FJ, Lopez Cillero P, Rufian Pena S, Solozano Peck G, Fugarolas G, Pera Madrazo C: Prospective and randomized study on the usefulness of octreotide in the prevention of complications after cephalic duodenopancreatectomy. Rev Esp Enferm Dig 1998;90:687–694.

20 Lowy AM, Lee JE, Pisters PWT, Davidson BS, Fenoglio CJ, Stanford P, Jinnah R, Evans DB: Prospective, randomized trial of octreotide to prevent pancreatic fistula after pancreaticoduodenectomy for malignant disease. Ann Surg 1997;226:632–641.

21 Fourtanier E, Chipponi J, Fagniez PL, Hay JM, Haddad AE, Fingerhut A: Octreotide in the prevention of surgical complications after pancreatectomy. A prospective randomized multicenter study. Hepatogastroenterology 1998;45(suppl): Abstract 429.

22 Friess H, Büchler M, Meschenmoser L, Dennler HJ, Malfertheiner P: Effect of octreotide on exocrine pancreatic function in man. Pancreas 1989;4:616.
23 Kemmer TP, Malfertheiner P, Büchler M, Friess H, Meschenmoser L, Ditschuneit H: Inhibition of human exocrine pancreatic secretion by the long-acting somatostatin analogue octreotide. Aliment Pharmacol Ther 1992;6:41–50.
24 Friess H, Bordihn K, Ebert M, Malfertheiner P, Kemmer T, Dennler HJ, Büchler MW: Inhibition of pancreatic secretion under long-term octreotide treatment in humans. Digestion 1994; 55:10–15.
25 Taparel D, Susini C, Esteve JR, Diaz J, Cazaubon C, Vaysse N, Ribet A: Somatostatin analogs: Correlation of receptor affinity with inhibition of cyclic AMP formation in pancreatic acinar cells. Peptides 1985;6:109–113.
26 Büchler MW, Binder M, Friess H: Role of somatostatin and its analogues in the treatment of acute and chronic pancreatitis. Gut 1994;3:15–19.
27 Starzl TE, Todo S, Tzakis A, Podesta L, Mieles L, Demetris A, Teperman L, Selby R, Stevenson W, Stieber A, Gordon R, Iwatsuki S: Abdominal organ cluster transplantation for the treatment of upper abdominal malignancies. Ann Surg 1989;210:374–386.
28 Daloze P, Beauregard H, St Louis G, Corman J, Smeesters C, Aris-Jilwain N, Comtois R, Rasio E: Clinical pancreas transplantation: A learning curve of its management. Transplant Proc 1989; 21:2858–2861.

Digestion

Digestion 1999;60(suppl 2):23–30

The Role of Octreotide and Somatostatin in Acute and Chronic Pancreatitis

W. Uhl S.E. Anghelacopoulos H. Friess M.W. Büchler

Department of Visceral and Transplantation Surgery, University of Bern, Switzerland

Key Words
Acute pancreatitis · Chronic pancreatitis · Pseudocyst · Fistula · Pancreatic ascites · Octreotide · Somatostatin · Conservative treatment

Abstract
Acute pancreatitis may follow a mild or a severe course. Whereas mild or edematous pancreatitis is a self-limiting disease with a low complication rate and low death rate, morbidity and mortality in severe or necrotizing pancreatitis are still unacceptably high. The major problem is the lack of a specific drug, especially in the early phase of the disease, to interfere with the systemic inflammatory response syndrome and to limit or prevent complications of the disease. Although the initiating pathophysiological process is not known, the destruction of the gland ('autodigestion') by digestive enzymes may be responsible for disease progression. Inhibition of pancreatic activity, which reduces exocrine secretion and further prevents the release and activation of enzymes, was therefore suggested as a specific treatment concept. The results of clinical investigations using somatostatin or its analogue are controversial, since all these trials had low statistical power. In a recent multicenter randomized controlled study with a large number of patients (n = 302) (and an adequate level of disease severity), no benefit of octreotide on progression or outcome was found. Chronic pancreatitis is characterized by an irreversible destruction of the exocrine and endocrine pancreatic parenchyma leading to maldigestion and diabetes. Pain, which may be caused by increased ductal pressure, is one of the most dominant symptoms in chronic pancreatitis. However, no beneficial effects on pain with pancreatic exocrine secretion-inhibiting drugs have been demonstrated. Treatment of other complications of the disease (pseudocyst formation, fistula and pancreatic ascites), with somatostatin or octreotide has given conflicting results. However, in a prophylactic clinical setting (e.g. elective pancreatic surgery) the inhibition of exocrine pancreatic secretion reduces complications.

Acute Pancreatitis

Up to 80% of patients with acute pancreatitis suffer from a mild and self-limiting disease which responds well to conservative treatment without any specific medication. Morphologically, this form of the disease is characterized by edema in and around the pancreas, and peripancreatic fatty tissue necrosis may occur. The other 20% of patients display a rapid, clinically severe course with pancreatic parenchymal and extrapancreatic necroses [1–3]. While both the complication and mortality rates in edematous acute pancreatitis are low (<1%), patients suffering from the necrotizing form develop systemic organ complications and have a mortality rate between 10–50% despite improved therapies [1, 4–7]. From a clinical point of view, the natural course of severe acute pancreatitis has two phases. The first, within 14 days of the onset of symptoms, is characterized by the necrosis of pancreatic parenchyma and peripancreatic

KARGER
Fax +41 61 306 12 34
E-Mail karger@karger.ch
www.karger.ch

0012–2823/99/0608–0023$17.50/0

Accessible online at:
http//BioMedNet.com/karger

Markus W. Büchler, MD
Chairman of the Department of Visceral and Transplantation Surgery
University Hospital of Bern, Inselspital CH–3010 Bern (Switzerland)
Tel. +41 31 632 2404, Fax +41 31 632 8552, E-Mail markus.buechler@insel.ch

fatty tissue. The generation and liberation of vasoactive and toxic substances and mediators cause a systemic inflammatory response syndrome (SIRS) which leads to lung, renal and cardiocirculatory organ dysfunction. The second phase (after 14 days) is associated with septic complications resulting from infected pancreatic necrosis [8–11].

Patients with severe acute pancreatitis should be placed in intensive care and treated with conservative therapeutic measures. At present, no single drug has been proven to interfere effectively with SIRS and thus limit or prevent further complications. To improve these unacceptably high rates of complications and mortality in severe acute pancreatitis, a specific treatment is urgently needed. Although the initiating pathophysiological processes are not known, the disease is caused by the destruction of the gland and peripancreatic fatty tissue by digestive enzymes [12–18]. These enzymes are produced in the acinar cells and activated in two possible ways (e.g. intra- and/or extracellularly). This 'autodigestion' process was suggested by Opie [17] in 1901. Furthermore, in experimental models of acute pancreatitis it has been demonstrated that the stimulation of exocrine pancreatic secretion leads to further deterioration. Therefore, the inhibition of pancreatic activity appears to be a reasonable first step in treatment. In order to interfere with the first phase of severe acute pancreatitis, two treatment options might be useful: (1) blockage or inhibition of activated enzymes by protease inhibitors or drugs targeting mediators, and (2) inhibition of exocrine pancreatic activity to prevent the release and activation of digestive enzymes. However, protease inhibitors (like aprotinin, gabexate mesylate) and hormones (like glucagon and somatostatin) have been investigated in human acute pancreatitis without success [4, 12–15].

Octreotide is a synthetic somatostatin analogue consisting of eight amino acids. In volunteers, it is a potent inhibitor of both basal and stimulated exocrine pancreatic secretion at a dose of 100 μg t.i.d. Further advantages of octreotide in comparison with the native hormone, somatostatin, are an increased half-life, higher potency, and subcutaneous application [19, 20]. The only limit to the use of octreotide in acute pancreatitis may be the reduction of splanchnic blood flow, since changes in microcirculation or hemodynamic properties can lead to further deterioration in the disease [21–23]. However, other authors found octreotide to protect against postischemic reperfusion injuries [24]. Furthermore, preliminary data suggest that octreotide, in contrast to somatostatin, increases the contractility of the sphincter of Oddi [25]. Both negative effects have not been seen in human acute pancreatitis.

Somatostatin and octreotide have been investigated in a number of experimental animal studies, with controversial results [26–31]. To explain the negative results, some reports suggested that basal and stimulated exocrine pancreatic secretion are reduced or almost abolished after the induction of acute pancreatitis [32, 33]. From these results it was concluded that the use of exocrine pancreatic secretion-inhibiting drugs does not influence the progression and outcome of the disease. In contrast to these findings in animal experiments, analysis of basal exocrine pancreatic secretion in humans revealed a normal secretory pattern during the acute inflammatory phase [34]. Additionally, it has been demonstrated that mRNA expression of pancreatic enzymes exists, indicating further enzyme synthesis following the induction of acute pancreatitis [35].

The first study of somatostatin in human acute pancreatitis was published in 1980 [36]. In 14 patients treated with somatostatin at a continuous intravenous dose of 250 μg/h for 3–4 days, the authors found 'an impressive clinical improvement in all patients'. Other controlled randomized trials of somatostatin in acute pancreatitis produced mixed results. A meta-analysis [37] taking into account all studies with an adequate study design revealed that the individual trials are clinically of poor discriminatory value due to low patient numbers and a lack of statistical power. The meta-analysis showed a significant reduction ($p < 0.01$) in mortality from 14% (29/207) in the placebo group to 6.2% (13/207) in the patient population receiving somatostatin.

A phase I–II study [38] of patients with moderate to severe acute pancreatitis treated with three different doses of octreotide (100, 200 and 500 μg t.i.d). showed a reduced incidence of new complications, especially at 200 μg t.i.d. Therefore, five rationales for the use octreotide in the treatment of acute pancreatitis were established: (1) a reduced mortality rate as shown by the meta-analysis of controlled randomized studies using the native hormone somatostatin [37]; (2) unchanged exocrine pancreatic secretion in the early phase of acute pancreatitis [34]; (3) the positive and promising results in an open phase I–II study using octreotide at a dose of 200 μg t.i.d. [38]; (4) the possible cyto- and organoprotective as well as stimulatory effect of somatostatin and its analogue on the RES [28–41], and (5) the continuation of pancreatic enzyme synthesis after the induction of the disease [35].

Table 1. Prospective clinical studies using somatostatin or its analogue octreotide in human acute pancreatitis

Group (first author)	Patients, n	Results, remarks
Mitrovic [43]	80	Significant reduction in complications and mortality by somatostatin
Gjorup [44]	63	No effect on complications and mortality; inclusion of mild disease
Luengo [45]	100	No effect on mortality; inclusion of mild disease
Beechey-Newman [46]	19	No effect on mortality; inclusion of mild disease
O'Hair [47]	180	Octreotide reduced complications; inclusion of mild disease
Paran [48]	38	Octreotide significantly reduced complications; open trial
Fiedler [49]	93	Octreotide significantly reduced mortality; open trial
McKay [50]	58	No effect of octreotide on complications and mortality; low number of cases
Uhl [42]	302	No effect of octreotide on complications and mortality

Clinical Trials with Somatostatin and Octreotide in Acute Pancreatitis [42–50]

Results from trials on somatostatin or octreotide in patients with acute pancreatitis are given in table 1. Three studies on the native hormone somatostatin reported conflicting results [43–45]. In 80 patients with severe acute pancreatitis, Mitrovic et al. [43] reported both a significant reduction in mortality from 40% (16/40) to 20% (8/40) and in complications including deaths from 58% (23/40) to 33% (13/40). In a double-blind, placebo-controlled multicenter trial by Gjorup et al. [44], the effect of continuous intravenous somatostatin infusion (250 µg/h for 3 days) was investigated in 63 patients suffering from acute pancreatitis. Although the patients were enrolled within 24 h of onset of symptoms, no significant benefit in terms of disease progression was found. No data were provided on the severity of disease at study entry. Based on the low mortality rate in this study (3%), it is assumed that only mild cases of acute pancreatitis were enrolled.

The other clinical studies investigating octreotide were published by Beechey-Newman [46], O'Hair et al. [47], Paran et al. [48], Fiedler et al. [49] and McKay et al. [50]. The first trial [46] investigated a high-dose treatment regimen consisting of an initial 250-µg subcutaneous octreotide bolus followed within 1 h by an intravenous infusion of 0.5 µg/kg/h for at least 10 days, in 19 patients. The octreotide group required significantly less analgesia ($p<0.05$), and developed fewer signs associated with poor prognosis, such as fall in hematocrit of >10% ($p<0.05$), serum albumin <32 g/l, calcium <2.0 mmol/l, and $pO_2<10$ kPa. Weekly CT scans showed a significant reduction in ascites and peripancreatic edema ($p<0.05$). Again, the majority of patients in this study suffered from mild acute pancreatitis, as only 3 patients had a Ranson score of 3 and Glasgow score of 2. The paper of Paran et al. [48] reported unusually positive results for octreotide treatment in a rather small patient population ($n=38$). Nineteen patients received subcutanous octreotide at a dose of 100 µg t.i.d. (as in the present study), and 19 patients received standard treatment. The patients had to have 3 or more Ranson points to be included in the study and the severity was assessed by CT scans. The findings from the imaging procedure were assessed according to the Ranson grading system, and 35/39 (90%) had grade C or more. These authors found significant decreases in septic complications (74 vs. 26%; $p=0.004$) and in the development of adult respiratory distress syndrome (ARDS) (63 vs. 18%; $p=0.02$), resulting in a significantly shorter hospital stay (34.1 vs. 17.9 days; $p=0.02$). As a main outcome variable, the mortality rate was lower in the group treated with octreotide, although the difference between groups was not statistically significant (37 vs. 11%; $p=0.1$).This study included patients with severe acute pancreatitis, but it can be criticized for the small number of patients and open-label design. Similar findings were reported by Fiedler et al. [49] in an open trial involving 39 patients with severe necrotizing acute pancreatitis. At a dose of 100 µg t.i.d., octreotide significantly reduced the frequency of ARDS (40 vs. 18 %; $p<0.05$), circulatory shock (87 vs. 51%; $p<0.05$) and mortality (26 vs. 61%; $p<0.01$). The results of this study must be interpreted with caution because the controls were 54 patients who were matched on a case-controlled basis from an earlier treatment period (1986–1992). Furthermore, contrary to current practice, all patients suffering from necrotizing acute pancreatitis underwent surgery. More recently published data by McKay et al. [50] from a small study (n = 58) with an adequate level of disease severity, found no significant differences in complications (54 vs. 40%) or mortality (18 vs. 20%).

The effect of octreotide on progression and outcome of acute pancreatitis in a double-blind, placebo-controlled, randomized, multicenter study was evaluated in a German-Swiss trial. The verum group consisted of two treatment arms with different octreotide doses, 100 µg t.i.d. (O100) and 200 µg t.i.d. (O200), while the control group received placebo. A total of 100 evaluable patients was planned for each group according to a power analysis. The first subcutanous injection was given immediately after enrollment. Further injections were administered at 8-hour intervals up to day 7 of the trial.

Patients with moderate to severe acute pancreatitis were enrolled in this study. Four obligatory and 4 out of 10 facultative inclusion criteria were defined. The obligatory criteria were: (1) first symptoms of acute pancreatitis within 4 days; (2) serum amylase or lipase more than three times the normal level within this time period; (3) upper abdominal pain during this time interval, and (4) written informed consent given to participate in the study. The ten facultative criteria were: (1) local abdominal resistance; (2) subileus/ileus; (3) circulatory shock: pulse rate $\leq$100/min and systolic blood pressure $\geq$80 mm Hg; (4) pO_2 <60 mm Hg; (5) leukocyte count >12,000/mm^3; (6) C-reactive protein >120 mg/l; (7) blood glucose >8.4 mmol/l (this criterion was not applied to known diabetics); (8) hypocalcemia <2.0 mmol/l; (9) serum creatinine >240 µmol/l, and (10) characteristic findings of moderate or severe acute pancreatitis in ultrasound or contrast-enhanced computed tomography.

Fifteen typical complications in acute pancreatitis were defined and assessed according to their clinical relevance: shock, sepsis, pulmonary and renal insufficiency, peritonitis, hemorrhage, infected necrosis/abscess, fluid collection, ileus/subileus, hypocalcemia, coagulation disorder, hyperglycemia, metabolic acidosis, jaundice and encephalopathy. These complications were followed during the treatment period daily until discharge. On the basis of these complications the severity of acute pancreatitis was assessed [for details, see 42].

This trial overcomes the limitations of the above-mentioned clinical studies. The study population is large (n = 302) and the severity of acute pancreatitis adequate, given the overall mortality rate of 16% (43/302) and the median Ranson and Apache II scores of 3 and 8, respectively. Despite sufficient statistical power, no clear positive ability of octreotide treatment to reduce complications and mortality in acute pancreatitis was found.

Table 2. Indications for octreotide in acute and chronic pancreatitis

Acute pancreatitis	–
Chronic pancreatitis	–
Prevention of complications after surgery	+
Prevention of complications after ERCP	?
Pancreatic pseudocyst	(+)
Fistula	(?+)

Nevertheless, octreotide can be helpful when given prior to trauma or operation as has been demonstrated in patients undergoing endoscopic retrograde cholangiopancreatography (ERCP) examination, pancreas transplantation or elective pancreatic surgery [51–59] (table 2). In patients with acute pancreatitis, however, there is rarely time for effective prophylactic measures. When the patient reaches hospital, it is often too late for treatment with specific drugs to prevent or ameliorate complications or SIRS in the early phase of severe disease. Once pancreatitis becomes acute, octreotide has been shown to have little effect on clinical outcome and progression of the disease. It appears that SIRS of severe acute pancreatitis can be managed successfully by maximum intensive care measures alone, without specific drugs. In view of the fact that septic complications remain the most important risk factor for death ($\geq$80%) and infections are common in the late phase of the disease, current drug treatment is targeted at the prevention of infected pancreatic necrosis. Early antibiotic therapy in patients with proven severe or necrotizing pancreatitis has been shown to reduce the infection rate of pancreatic necrosis and to delay the need for surgical intervention. Furthermore, due to the late infection, operative intervention is postponed to the third or fourth week after onset of symptoms with then optimal surgical condition for necrosectomy of good demarcated pancreatic necrosis [5, 10, 11, 60].

Chronic Pancreatitis

Chronic pancreatitis is an irreversible disease of the exocrine pancreatic parenchyma. Recent advances in molecular and cellular biology have generated a better understanding of the disease [1, 61–65]. Histologically, it is characterized by a progressive inflammatory process with irreversible pathological changes leading to both exocrine and, in the late stages, endocrine pancreatic insufficiency [66]. Histopathological changes involve different degrees of fibrosis, atrophy of acinar cells in tubular structures, and infiltration of the parenchyma by inflammatory cells. Alcohol abuse is the major etiological factor in chronic pancreatitis, accounting for 70–80% of cases. Additional predisposing causes include cholelithiasis, pancreatic duct obstruction and hereditary factors [67–70].

Despite recent intensive research, the pathophysiology of chronic pancreatitis remains uncertain since none of the different accepted pathophysiological concepts can fully explain the morphological and histological alterations that occur. Four hypotheses have been proposed as the most important pathomechanisms of chronic pancreatitis: (1) according to Sarles et al. [71], chronic alcohol intake causes a qualitative change in pancreatic secretion, with formation of protein plugs and calcification in the ductal system of the pancreatic gland. The formation of calcium crystals is due to a decreased expression of lithostatin, a calcium stabilizer. The obstruction of the pancreatic duct system induces chronic inflammation with atrophy of pancreatic acinar cells and fibroblastic proliferation. (2) Recurrent attacks of acute pancreatitis lead to small areas of interstitial fat necrosis and hemorrhage followed by perilobular fibrosis and duct obstruction. (3) Oxidative stress is caused by increased levels of free radicals and disorders in hepatic detoxification. (4) Finally, direct toxic effects of ethanol and its metabolites on the pancreatic parenchyma are considered to play an important role in the pathophysiology of chronic pancreatitis [72–74]. Recently, it has been reported that growth factors (EGF, TGF) and growth factor receptors (c-erB-2 proto-oncogene) may play a role in the pathobiological mechanisms that occur in chronic pancreatitis and contribute to interstitial fibrosis [75, 76].

The most common symptom of chronic pancreatitis is abdominal pain which can range from mild discomfort to disabling pain requiring the use of narcotics [77]. The disease is often complicated by pancreatic pseudocysts, with reported incidences of 40–60% [78]. Regardless of size, these require interventional/surgical therapy if they do not respond to conservative treatment. Pancreatic ascites and pleural effusion by fistula are rarely associated with chronic pancreatitis. These complications are usually managed conservatively, with therapeutic regimens selected on the basis of thorough examinations including CT/MRI and ERCP findings [1, 65].

The effects of somatostatin or octreotide on the above complications resulting from pancreatic exocrine secretion have been investigated in several studies [79–95]. Both drugs appear to be effective in some cases (table 2).

Intractable Pain in Chronic Pancreatitis

It has been suggested that pancreatic ductal hypertension due to outflow obstruction is the major cause of pain in chronic pancreatitis, while other causes may be blood flow alteration, inflammatory involvement of intrapancreatic nerves, or complications of the disease itself (e.g. pseudocysts or compression of adjacent visceral structures) [65, 81]. In an open trial of somatostatin in 15 patients with chronic pancreatitis and recurrent abdominal pain, Loginov et al. [83] found pain relief in all cases. Based on the positive results with octreotide seen in another study, Toskes [84] concluded that this drug may become an important therapy for abdominal pain unresponsive to pancreatic enzyme therapy. These effects, however, were not confirmed in a previously published trial. In an intraindividual, double-blind, placebo-controlled crossover study of 10 patients with chronic pancreatitis, Malfertheiner et al. [85] investigated the effect of octreotide (100 μg/day t.i.d.) for 3 days. Pancreatic secretion was monitored daily by measuring fecal chymotrypsin concentration. The authors found that during the administration of octreotide, pancreatic secretion was strongly inhibited (octreotide vs. placebo: mean fecal chymotrypsin 1.7 vs. 9.6 U/g; $p < 0.001$). However, pain score and consumption of analgesics were not different during the octreotide and placebo periods. It was concluded that short-term inhibition of pancreatic secretion does not result in pain relief in patients with chronic pancreatitis.

Pseudocysts and Fistula in Chronic Pancreatitis

Pancreatic pseudocysts are a common and painful complication in chronic pancreatitis. The mechanisms which cause pseudocyst formation are not yet fully understood. Pseudocysts following an acute pancreatitis have a different pathogenesis from those arising during the course of chronic inflammatory disease [86, 87]. Pseudocysts in chronic pancreatitis are caused by the obstruction of the pancreatic duct system leading to an increase in intraductal pressure and a localized rupture of the main pancreatic duct and its trees. Extravasation of pancreatic fluid is thereafter walled off by inflammatory fibrosis leading to the formation of the pseudocyst. Adams and Anderson [88] published accounts of their 27 years of experience in the surgical management of 160 patients with pancreatic pseudocysts. The authors recommended the use of octreotide for persistent pancreatic fistula. Barkin et al. [89] studied the adjuvant role of octreotide in the management of 3 patients with pancreatic pseudocysts who had prolonged catheter drainage. It was shown that octreotide decreased persistent drainage from chronic pancreatic pseudocyst. Similar findings were reported by Gullo and Barbara [90] from a slightly larger clinical trial. In 4 out of 7 patients, pain disappeared and pseudocyst decreased in size. D'Agostino et al. [91] used a combined regimen of percutaneous drainage and administration of octreotide in patients with symptomatic pseudocyst and chronic pancreatitis. This treatment was successful in 7 out of 8 cases, and the authors concluded that octreotide effectively decreases the output from pancreatic pseudocysts drained percutaneously. However, further randomized controlled clinical trials are urgently needed before somatostatin and its analogue should be recommended in the treatment of pain or therapy of pseudocyst and pancreatic fistula in patients with chronic pancreatitis.

References

1 Büchler MW, Uhl W, Malfertheiner P (eds): Pankreaserkrankungen: Akute Pankreatitis, Chronische Pankreatitis, Pankreastumore. Basel, Karger, 1996.
2 Beger HG, Bittner R, Büchler M, Hess W, Schmitz JE: Hemodynamic data pattern in patients with acute pancreatitis. Gastroenterology 1986;90:74–79.
3 Isenmann R, Büchler M, Uhl W, Martini M, Beger HG: Pancreatic necrosis is an early finding in severe acute pancreatitis. Pancreas 1993; 8:358–361.
4 Leese T, Holliday M, Watkins M, Neoptolemos JP, Thomas WM, Attard A. A multicentre controlled clinical trial of high-volume fresh-frozen plasma therapy in prognostically severe acute pancreatitis. Ann R Coll Surg Engl 1991;73: 207–214.
5 Luiten EJT, Hop WCJ, Lanje JF, Bruining HA: Controlled clinical trial of selective decontamination for the treatment of severe acute pancreatitis. Ann Surg 1995;222:57–65.
6 Rattner DW, Legermate DA, Lee MJ, Mueller PR, Warshaw A: Surgical debridement of symptomatic pancreatic necrosis is beneficial irrespective of infection. Am J Surg 1992;163: 105–110.
7 Sainio V, Kemppainen E, Puolakkainen P, Taavitsainen M, Kivisaari L, Valtonen V, Haapiainen R, Schröder T, Kivilaakso E: Early antibiotic treatment in acute necrotising pancreatitis. Lancet 1995;346:663–667.
8 Uhl W, Büchler M, Malfertheiner P, Martini M, Beger HG: PMN-elastase in comparison with CRP, antiproteases and LDH as indicators of necrosis in human acute pancreatitis. Pancreas 1991;6:253–259.
9 Uhl W, Schrag HJ, Schmitter N, Nevalainen TJ, Aufenanger J, Wheatley AM, Büchler MW: The pathophysiological role of secretory type I and II phospholipase A_2 in acute pancreatitis. An experimental study in the rat. Gut 1997;40:386–392.
10 Beger HG, Bittner R, Block S, Büchler M: Bacterial contamination of pancreatic necrosis. A prospective study. Gastroenterology 1986;91: 433–438.
11 Uhl W, Büchler MW. The role of surgery in pancreatic sepsis. Dig Surg 1996;13:374–380.
12 Büchler M, Malfertheiner P, Uhl W, Schölmerich J, Stöckmann F, Adler G, Gaus W, Rolle K, Beger HG: Gabexate mesylate in human acute pancreatitis. Gastroenterology 1993;104:1165–1170.
13 Regan PT, Malagelada JR, Go VLW, Wolf AM, DiMagno EP: A prospective study of cimetidine and glucagon in human acute pancreatitis. Mayo Clin Proc 1981;56:499–503.
14 Schmid St, Uhl W, Büchler MW: Protease-antiprotease interactions and the rationale for therapeutic protease inhibitors. Scand J Gastroenterol 1996;219:47–50.
15 Steinberg WM, Schlesselmann SE: Treatment of acute pancreatitis: Comparison of animal and human studies. Gastroenterology 1987;93:1420–1427.
16 Adler G, Kern HF, Scheele GA: Experimental models and concepts of acute pancreatitis; in Go VLW, Gardner JD, Brooks FP, et al: The Exocrine Pancreas. New York, Raven Press, 1986, pp 407–421.
17 Opie EL: The etiology of acute hemorrhagic pancreatitis. Bull John Hopkins 1901;12:182–18.
18 Uhl W, Isenmann R, Curti G, Vogel R, Beger HG, Büchler MW: Influence of the etiology on the course and outcome of acute pancreatitis. Pancreas 1996;13:335–343.
19 Bauer W, Briner U, Doepfner WW, Haller R, Huguenin R, Marbach P, Petcher TJ, Pless J: SMS 201-995: A very potent and selective octapeptide analogue of somatostatin with prolonged action. Life Sci 1982;31:1133–1140.
20 Kemmer TP, Malferteiner P, Büchler M, Friess H, Meschenmoser L, Ditschuneit H: Inhibition of human exocrine pancreatic secretion by the long-acting somatostatin analogue octreotide (SMS 201-995). Aliment Pharmacol Ther 1992; 6:41–50.
21 Herzog L, Ryschich E, Schmidt J, Gebhard MM, Herfarth C, Klar E: Octreotide reduces blood flow in ischemic areas of the pancreas in acute pancreatitis. Langenbecks Arch Chir Suppl Kongressbd 1997;114:407–411.
22 Mastai R, Bosch J, Navasa M, Rodes J: Effect of continuous and bolus injections of somatostatin on azygos blood flow and hepatic and system haemodynamics in patients with portal hypertension: Comparison with vasopressin. J Hepatol 1986;3:A53.
23 Sonnenberg GE, Keller U, Purruchud D, Gyr K: Effect of somatostatin on splanchnic haemodynamics in patients with cirrhosis of the liver and in normal subjects. Gastroenterology 1981; 80:526–532.
24 Hoffmann TF, Uhl E, Messmer K: Protective effect of the somatostatin analogue octreotide in ischemic/reperfusion-induced acute pancreatitis in rats. Pancreas 1996;12:286–293.
25 DiFrancesco V, Angelini G, Bovo P, Casarini MB, Filippini M, Vaona B, Frulloni L, Rigo L, Brunori MP, Cavallini G: Effect of octreotide on sphincter of Oddi motility in patients with acute recurrent pancreatitis: A manometric study. Dig Dis Sci 1996;41:2392–2396.
26 Augelli NV, Hussain SM, McKain MM, Fietsam R, Bierema T, Fegley M, Bendick P, Villalba M, Lucas R, Glover JL: Effect of MS 201-995 (a long-acting somatostatin analog) on bile-induced acute hemorrhagic pancreatitis in the dog. Arch Surg 1989;55:389–391.
27 Baxter JN, Jenkins SA, Day DW, Roberts NB, Cowell DC, Mackie CR, Shields R: Effects of somatostatin and a long-acting somatostatin analogue on the prevention and treatment of experimentally induced acute pancreatitis. Br J Surg 1985;72:382–385.
28 Baxter JN, Jenkins SA, Day DW, Shields R: Effects of a somatostatin analogue on hepatic and splenic reticulo-endothelial function in rats. Br J Surg 1985;75:1005–1008.
29 Jenkins SA, Baxter JN, Day DW, Al-Sumidaie AM, Leinster SJ, Shields R: The effects of somatostatin and SMS 201-995 on experimentally-induced pancreatitis and endotoxemia with cirrhosis and portal hypertension. Klin Wochenschr 1986;64:100–1006
30 Schwedes U, Althoff PH, Klempa I, Leushner U, Mothes L, Raptis S, et al: Effect of somatostatin on bile-induced acute hemorrhagic pancreatitis in the dog. Horm Metab Res 1979;11: 655–661.

31 Zhu ZH, Holt S, El-Lbishi MS, Grady T, Taylor TV, Powers RE: A somatostatin analogue is protective against retrograde bile salt-induced pancreatitis in the rat. Pancreas 1991;6:609–613.
32 Evander A, Hederström E, Hultberg B, Ihse I: Exocrine pancreatic secretion in acute experimental pancreatitis. Digestion 1982;24:159–167.
33 Niederau C, Niederau M, Lüthen R, Strohmeyer G, Ferrell LD, Grendel JH: Pancreatic exocrine secretion in acute experimental pancreatitis. Gastroenterology 1990;99:1120–1127.
34 Dominguez-Munoz JE, Pieramico O, Büchler M, Malfertheiner P: Exocrine pancreatic function in the early phase of human acute pancreatitis. Scand J Gastroenterol 1995;30:186–191.
35 Uhl W, Friess H, Häggblom JO, Riesle E, Deflorin J, Büchler MW: Die Expression von Pankreasenzymen ist in der Fühphase der experimentellen akuten Pankreatitis nicht aufgehoben – Eine Therapieoption für Sekretionshemmer. Langenbeck Arch Chir Suppl Chir Forum 1996;477–481.
36 Limberg K, Kommerell B: Treatment of acute pancreatitis with somatostatin. N Engl J Med 1980;79:284.
37 Carballo F, Dominguez-Munoz JE, Fernandez-Calvet L, Martinez-Pancorbo C, Garcia A, de la Morena J: Is somatostatin useful in the treatment of acute pancreatitis? A meta-analysis. Digestion 1991;49:A12–13.
38 Binder M, Uhl W, Friess H, Malfertheiner P, Büchler MW: Octreotide in the treatment of acute pancreatitis: Results of a unicenter prospective trial with three different octreotide dosages. Digestion 1994;55:20–23.
39 Eliakin R, Karmeli F, Okon E, Rachmilewitz D: Octreotide effectively deceases mucosal damage in experimental colitis. Gut 1993;34:264–269.
40 Szabo S, Usadel KH: Cytoprotection-organoprotection by somatostatin: Gastric and hepatic lesions. Experientia 1982;38:254–256.
41 Usadel KH, Kessler H, Rohr G, Kusterer K, Palitzsch KD, Schwedes U: Cytoprotective properties of somatostatins. Klin Wochenschr 1986;64(suppl 7):59–63.
42 Uhl W, Büchler MW, Malfertheiner P, Beger HG, Adler G, Gaus W, and the German Pancreatitis Study Group: A randomized, double-blind, multicenter trial of octreotide in moderate to severe acute pancreatitis. Gut 1999; in press.
43 Mitrovic M, Sijacid A, Todoravim M, Karamarkovic A: Acute pancreatitis treated with somatostatin – The double-blind study. Proc Gastro-Surgical Club, Madrid 1993, pp 144–145.
44 Gjorup I, Roikjaer O, Andersen B, Burckarth F, Hovendal C, Pedersen SA, Christiansen P, Wara P, Andersen JC, Balsler I, Jepsen J, Rokkjaer M: A double-blinded multicenter trial of somatostatin in the treatment of acute pancreatitis. Surg Gynecol Obstet 1992;175:397–400.
45 Luengo L, Vicente V, Gris F, Coronas JM, Escuder J, Gomez JR, Castellote JM: Influence of somatostatin in the evolution of acute pancreatitis – A prospective randomized study. Int J Pancreatol 1994;15:139–144.
46 Beechey-Newman N: Controlled trial of high-dose octreotide in treatment of acute pancreatitis. Dig Dis Sci 1993;38:644–647.
47 O'Hair DP, Hoffmann RG, Schroeder H, Wilson SD: Octreotide in the treatment of acute pancreatitis: A prospective, randomized trial. Gastroenterology 1993;104:A326.
48 Paran H, Neufeld D, Mayo A, Shwartz J, Singer P, Kaplan O, Skornik Y, Klausner J, Freund U: Preliminary report of a prospective randomized study of octreotide in the treatment of severe acute pancreatitis. J Am Coll Surg 1995;181:121–124.
49 Fiedler F, Jauernig G, Keim V, Richter A, Bender HJ: Octreotide treatment in patients with necrotizing pancreatitis and pulmonary failure. Intensive Care Med 1996;22:909–915.
50 McKay C, Baxter J, Imrie C: A randomized, controlled trial of octreotide in the management of patients with acute pancreatitis. Int J Pancreatol 1997;21:13–19.
51 Binmoeller KF, Harris AG, Dumas R, Grimaldi C, Delmont JP: Does the somatostatin analogue octreotide protect against ERCP induced pancreatitis. Gut 1992;33:1129–1133.
52 Bordas JM, Toledo V, Mondelo F, Rodes J: Prevention of pancreatic reactions by bolus somatostatin administration in patients undergoing endoscopic retrograde cholangio-pancreatography and endoscopic sphincterotomy. Hormone Res 1988;29:106–108.
53 Büchler M, Friess H, Klempa I, Hermanek P, Sulkowski U, Becker H, Schafmayer A, Baca I, Lorenz D, Meister R, Kremes B, Wagner P, Witte J, Zurmayer EL, Jaeger HD, Rieck B, Dollinger P, Glaser K, Teichmann R, Konradt J, Gauss W, Dennler HF, Welzel D, Beger HG: The role of somatostatin analogue octreotide in the prevention of postoperative complications following pancreatic resection. The results of a multicenter controlled trial. Am J Surg 1992; 163:125–130.
54 Friess H, Beger HG, Sulkowski U, Becker H, Hofbauer B, Dennler HJ, Büchler MW: Randomized controlled multicentre study of the prevention of complications by octreotide in patients undergoing surgery for chronic pancreatitis. Br J Surg 1995;82:1270–1273.
55 Montorsi M, Zago M, Mosca F, Capussotti L, Zotti E, Ribotta G, Fegiz G, Fissi S, Roviaro G, Peracchia A, Pivi M, Perego R, Pezzuoli G: Efficacy of octreotide in the prevention of pancreatic fistula after elective pancreatic resections: A prospective, controlled, randomized clinical trial. Surgery 1995;117:26–31.
56 Pederzoli P, Bassi C, Falconi M, Camboni MG and the Italian Study Group: Efficacy of octreotide in the prevention of complications of elective pancreatic surgery. Br J Surg 1994;81:265–269.
57 Sternlieb JM, Aronchick CA, Retig JN, Dabezies M, Saunders F, Goosenberg E, Infantolino A, Ionna S, Maislin G, Wright SH: A multicenter, controlled trial to evaluate the effect of prophylactic octreotide on ERCP-induced pancreatitis. Am J Gastroenterol 1992;87:1561–1566.
58 Testoni PA, Lella F, Bagnolo F, Caporuscio S, Cattani L, Colombo E, Buizza M: Long-term prophylactic administration of octreotide reduces the rise in serum amylase after endoscopic procedures on Vater's papilla. Pancreas 1996; 13:61–65.
59 Benedetto E, Coady NT, Asolati M, Dunn T, Stormoen BM, Bartholomew AM, Vasquez EM, Pollak R: A prospective randomized clinical trial of perioperative treatment with octreotide in pancreas transplantation. Am J Surg 1998;175:14–17.
60 Pederzoli P, Bassi C, Vesentini S, Campedelli A: A randomized multicenter clinical trial of antibiotic prophylaxis of septic complications in acute necrotizing pancreatitis with imipenem. Surg Gynecol Obstet 1993;176:480–483.
61 DiMagno EP, Layer P, Clain JE: Chronic pancreatitis; in Go VLW, DiMagno EP, Gardner JD, Lebenthal E, Reber HA, Scheele GA (eds): The Exocrine Pancreas: Biology, Pathology, and Diseases. New York, Raven Press, 1993, pp 665–706.
62 Kashiwagi M, Friess H, Uhl W, Graber H, Duarte R, Zimmermann A, Büchler MW: Phospholipase A_2 isoforms are altered in chronic pancreatitis. Ann Surg 1998;227:220–228.
63 Di Sebastiano P, Fink T, Beger HG, Büchler MW: Immune cell infiltration and growth-associated protein-43 expression correlate with pain in chronic pancreatitis. Gastroenterology 1997; 112:1648–1652.
64 DiMagno EP: A short, elective history of exocrine pancreatic insufficiency and chronic pancreatitis. Gastroenterology 1993;104:1255–1262.
65 Dervenis CH, Friess H, Uhl W: Complications in chronic pancreatitis. Dig Surg 1996;13:79–89.
66 Bradley EI III: Complications in chronic pancreatitis. Surg Clin North Am 1989;69:481–497.
67 Srles H: Proposal adopted unanimously by the participants of the Symposium on Pancreatitis, Marseilles 1963. Bibl Gastroenterol 1965;7:VII–VIII.
68 Sarner M, Cotton PB: Pancreatitis – Concepts and classification. Gut 1984;25:756–759.
69 Singer MV, Gyr K, Sarles H: Revised classification of pancreatitis. Gastroenterology 1985;89: 683–685.
70 Sarles H, Adler G, Dani R, Frey L, Gullo L, Harada H, Martin E, Norohna M, Scuro LA: The pancreatitis classification of Marseilles, Rome 1988. Scand J Gastroenterol 1983;24: 651–652.
71 Sarles H, Bernard JP, Johnson C, Chir M: Pathogenesis and epidemiology of chronic pancreatitis. Annu Rev Med 1989;40:453–468.
72 Klöppel G, Maillet B: Pseudocysts in chronic pancreatitis: A morphological analysis of 57 resection specimens and 9 autopsy pancreata. Pancreas 1991;6:266–274.
73 Braganza JM: Pancreatic disease: A causality of hepatic 'detoxification'? Lancet 1983;ii:1000–1003.
74 Bordalo O, Bapista A, Dreiling D, Noronha M: Early pathomorphological pancreatic changes in chronic alcoholism; in Gyr KE, Singer MV, Sarles H (eds): Pancreatitis – Concepts and Classification. Amsterdam, Elsevier/North-Holland, 1982, No 642.

75 Bockman DE, Merlino G: Cytological changes in the pancreas of transgenic mice overexpressing transforming growth factor α. Gastroenterology 1992;103:1883–1892.

76 Korc M, Friss H, Yamanaka Y, Kobrin MS, Büchler MW, Beger HG: Chronic pancreatitis is associated with increased concentrations of epidermal growth factor receptor, trasforming growth factor alpha, and phospholipase C gamma. Gut 1994;35:1468–1473.

77 Veness JA: Chronic pancreatitis (editorial). Gastroenterology 1982;82:1471–1472.

78 Radun D, Malfertheiner P: Chronic pancreatitis: Conservative therapy. Ther Umsch 1995; 53:359–364.

79 Segal I, Parekh D, Lipschitz J, Gecelter G, Myburgh JA: Treatment of pancreatic ascites and external pancreatic fistulas with a long-acting somatostatin analogue. Digestion 1993; 54(suppl 1):53–58.

80 Kozarek RA, Traverso LW: Pancreatic fistulas: Etiology, consequences, and treatment. Gastroenterologist 1996;4:238–244.

81 Dominguez-Munoz JE, Malfertheiner P: Standards and limitations of conservative treatment in chronic pancreatitis. Dig Surg 1996;13:73–78.

82 Büchler MW, Binder M, Friss H: Role of somatostatin and its analogues in the treatment of acute and chronic pancreatitis. Gut 1994; 35(suppl):S15–S19.

83 Loginov AS, Sadokov VM, Vinokurova LV, Chernoiarova OD, Astafeva OV, Nilova TV: Atrial of the use of Sandostatin in patients with chronic pancreatitis. Ter Arkh 1995;67:60–62.

84 Toskes PP: Medical management of chronic pancreatitis. Scand J Gastroenterol 1995;208(suppl): 74–80.

85 Malfertheiner P, Mayer D, Büchler MW, Dominguez-Munoz JE, Shiefer B, Ditshuneit H: Treatment of pain in chronic pancreatitis by inhibition of pancreatic secretion with octreotide. Gut 1995;36:450–454.

86 Bradley EI, Clements JL, Gonzales AC: The natural history of pancreatic pseudocyst: A unified concept of management. Am J Surg 1979; 137:135–141.

87 McConnell DB, Gregory JR, Saski TM, Vetto RML: Pancreatic pseudocysts. Am J Surg 1982; 143:599–601.

88 Adams DB, Anderson MC: Changing concepts in the surgical management of pancreatic pseudocysts. Am Surg 1992;58:173–180

89 Barkin JS, Reiner DK, Deutch E: Sandostatin for control of catheter drainage of pancreatic pseudocyst. Pancreas 1991;6:245–248.

90 Gullo L, Barbara L: Treatment of pancreatic pseudocysts with octreotide. Lancet 1991;31: 540–541.

91 D'Agostino HB, van Sonnenberg E, Sanchez RB, Goodacre BW, Villaveiran RG, Lyche K: Treatment of pancreatic pseudocyst with percutaneous drainage and octreotide. Radiology 1993;187:685–688.

92 Nubiola-Calonge P, Badia JM, Sancho J, Gil MJ, Segura M, Sitges-Serra A: Blind evaluation of the effect of octreotide (SMS 201-995), a somatostatin analogue, on small-bowel fistula output. Lancet 1987;19:672–674.

93 Scott NA, Finnegan S, Irving MH: Octreotide and postoperative enterocutaneous fistulae: A controlled prospective study. Acta Gastroenterol Belg 1993;56:266–270.

94 Sancho JJ, Di Costanzo J, Nubiola P, Larrad A, Beguiristain A, Roqueta F, Franch G, Oliva A, Gubern JM, Sitges-Serra A: Randomized double-blind placebo-controlled trial of early octreotide in patients with postoperative enterocutaneous fistula. Br J Surg 1995;82:638–641.

95 Sitges-Serra A, Guirao X, Pereira JA, Nubiola P: Treatment of gastrointestinal fistulas with Sandostatin. Digestion 1993;54:38–40.

Digestion

Digestion 1999;60(suppl 2):31–41

Somatostatin or Octreotide in Acute Variceal Bleeding

Antoine Hadengue

Division of Gastroenterology and Hepatology, Hôpital Cantonal, Geneva, Switzerland

Key Words

Portal hypertension · Esophageal varices · Variceal bleeding · Somatostatin · Octreotide

Abstract

In patients with cirrhosis, somatostatin or octreotide administration is followed by a transient decrease in the hepatic venous pressure gradient and azygos blood flow. Although no clear-cut changes in variceal pressure are observed and the exact mechanisms of acute hemodynamic changes induced by somatostatin or its derivatives are still unknown, this provided the rationale for its use in patients with variceal hemorrhage. The only known sustained hemodynamic effect of octreotide is to prevent increases in hepatic venous gradient or azygos blood flow in response to food intake.

Somatostatin infusion can be as effective as sclerotherapy in the initial control of bleeding esophageal varices in patients with cirrhosis and is associated with fewer complications. Octreotide also seems to be as effective as endoscopic therapy in the control of acute variceal bleeding, although larger studies should be performed before its efficacy and safety profile can be fully evaluated.

The combination of somatostatin or long-acting analogues to endoscopic therapy has recently been delineated as one of the most promising approaches in these patients. Early somatostatin administration with repeat boluses, starting several hours before sclerotherapy is combined, eases the endoscopic procedure and reduces bleeding control failure rate. Although two studies also showed that octreotide, when started at the time of sclerotherapy or variceal banding, also improves bleeding control, a conclusion on octreotide use in these patients is premature. Optimal administration schedules and doses of somatostatin or octreotide are still unknown. The safety of octreotide in patients with variceal bleeding, which has recently been challenged, should be assessed in larger trials.

Recent data suggesting that octreotide combination to β-blockers or sclerotherapy may represent a useful approach for long-term prevention of rebleeding in these patients will have to be confirmed.

Background

Between 50 and 60% of patients with cirrhosis will develop gastroesophageal varices. Thirty percent of these will experience variceal bleeding within 2 years. Thirty percent of those who bleed will eventually die in relation to the bleeding episode [1, 2]. Adequate care for an acute bleeding episode includes the early administration of vasoactive drugs that may arrest the hemorrhage and ease diagnostic endoscopy, management by a trained gastrointestinal bleeding team, and mandatory endoscopy with the possibility to offer sclerotherapy or banding.

Four vasoactive drugs, vasopressin, terlipressin, somatostatin and octreotide, have been shown to achieve some efficacy in the control of acute variceal hemorrhage. Because it can induce severe side effects, and is less efficacious than terlipressin or somatostatin [3], the use of vasopressin has now been abandoned in Europe. Terlipressin is more effective and results in fewer side effects

KARGER

Fax +41 61 306 12 34
E-Mail karger@karger.ch
www.karger.ch

0012–2823/99/0608–0031$17.50/0

Accessible online at:
http//BioMedNet.com/karger

Antoine Hadengue
Division de Gastroentérologie et d'Hépatologie
Hopital Cantonal
CH–1211 Genève (Switzerland)
Tel. +4122 372 9340, Fax +4122 372 9366, E-Mail antoine.hadengue@hcuge.ch

than vasopressin. Four recent trials compared somatostatin or octreotide to terlipressin alone [4–6] or associated with nitroglycerin [7]. All four concluded that terlipressin was comparable to somatostatin or octreotide for the control of bleeding. However, in two of these studies [5, 6], side effects were significantly more frequent with terlipressin than somatostatin or octreotide. A third study [7], although it did not demonstrate a statistically significant difference in the incidence of side effects, reported severe bradycardia due to terlipressin in 2 patients, which was responsible for death in 1. This review will focus on the results of controlled studies with somatostatin or octreotide in the management of acute bleeding in these patients. The comparison of somatostatin or its derivatives with terlipressin, which has been briefly summarized above, will not be further discussed. Finally, since balloon tamponade is only used as a salvage procedure, not as a first-line choice, comparisons with tamponade will not be mentioned in this review.

Three major trends have emerged during the 1990s in delineating the use of drugs in the emergency treatment of upper gastrointestinal bleeding in patients with cirrhosis. First, the Baveno international consensus workshop provided clear statements on definitions, diagnostic evaluation, and methodological requirements for trials in patients with portal hypertension [8]. These definitions and requirements should not only guide future trials but also help in the analysis of previously published studies. Second, the concept of early pharmacological therapy for gastroesophageal bleeding has become accepted as part of first-line management. Its evaluation should take into account (a) the early control of the variceal bleed; (b) the prevention of rebleeding which occurs in 30–50% of the patients within the 6 weeks that follow an index bleed, and (c) mortality at 6 weeks which is usually related to the deterioration of liver function following variceal bleeding. Third, while the question remained for a long time 'Does pharmacological do better than endoscopic treatment?', it is becoming 'Does early drug administration help patients who eventually will receive endoscopic therapy?'

Somatostatin and Its Analogues

Somatostatin is a natural peptide, which is secreted by pancreatic islet D cells and cells disseminated throughout the intestinal tract with the highest density in the antrum and duodenum. Preprosomatostatin, a 166-amino-acid protein encoded by chromosome 3, is processed to biologically active somatostatin 28 or 14. Somatostatin 14, the therapeutic compound, has a half-life of 2–3 min. Inhibition by somatostatin of the secretion of a number of hormones thought to play a role in the maintenance of portal hypertension (including glucagon and VIP) initially provided the rationale for its use in patients with esophageal varices.

Octreotide is a synthetic cyclic octapeptide that shares four essential amino acids with somatostatin. Its half-life is longer than that of somatostatin, and may be as long as 4 h in patients with cirrhosis [9]. While somatostatin binds to all five human somatostatin receptors (SSTR 1 to 5), octreotide essentially binds to subtypes 2 and 5, with intermediate binding to subtype 3 and no binding to other subtypes [10]. It is conceivable that, due to this specificity of octreotide for some, not all somatostatin receptors, differences may exist between octreotide and somatostatin hemodynamic effects.

Many other analogues of somatostatin have been developed, some of which are currently investigated for possible use in patients with portal hypertension [for a review, see 10].

Hemodynamic Effects of Somatostatin or Octreotide in Patients with Cirrhosis

Systemic, splanchnic and renal effects of somatostatin or octreotide seem to vary according to the dose and, mostly, to the mode of administration, i.e. bolus or continuous infusion.

After a bolus infusion of somatostatin [11] or octreotide [12] in stable patients with cirrhosis, an immediate systemic vasoconstrictor effect was observed, while in most studies continuous infusion was not associated with systemic hemodynamic changes. In the study by McCormick et al. [12] the response to octreotide bolus infusion (25 μg, IV) was characterized by immediate and transient elevation in mean arterial pressure (from 81 to 87 mm Hg) and mean pulmonary pressures (from 9.1 to 16.6 mm Hg) together with a reduction in pulse rate (from 77 to 65 beats/min) and cardiac output (from 9.2 to 7.9 l/min). These effects promptly disappeared a few minutes after bolus administration and were less marked during continuous infusion at a dose of 50 μg/h [12]. Thus, in stable patients with cirrhosis, octreotide appears to correct, in a transient manner, the systemic hyperkinetic circulation.

Similarly, somatostatin 250 μg bolus administration markedly but transiently decreases the hepatic venous pressure gradient (HVPG). This was evaluated in a double-blind hemodynamic study by Cirera et al. [13]

who demonstrated an HVPG reduction of 52% at 1 min, 19% at 3 min and 13% at 5 min. Azygos blood flow (ABF) also decreased by 45% at 1 min, 16% at 3 min, and 9.5% at 5 min. However, continuous 250 μg/h somatostatin infusion was associated with only marginal or no change in the HVPG or ABF, respectively [13]. Increasing the dose of somatostatin to 500 μg/h achieved a 23% decrease in ABF [13]. In a double-blind controlled study [14], we compared the hemodynamic effects of octreotide (25 μg bolus followed by 25 μg//h infusion), somatostatin (250 μg bolus followed by 250μg/h infusion) or placebo. ABF significantly decreased 5–15 min after octreotide or somatostatin, but had returned to baseline 60 min after octreotide. Furthermore, it was evidenced that 60 min after somatostatin, ABF in fact increased to values above baseline, suggesting the occurrence of a rebound phenomenon [14].

The question of variceal pressure changes after somatostatin or octreotide infusion remains controversial. While most authors failed to document significant changes [15, 16], some showed transient decreases or even increases in variceal pressure [17]. It can be noted that the methods used to measure variceal pressure, as well as the doses of somatostatin or octreotide used, greatly varied from one study to another. In a recent work, Barrioz et al. [18] evidenced a marked and sustained increase in lower esophageal sphincter pressure after octreotide administration in patients with cirrhosis and speculated this might participate in the effect of octreotide on esophageal varices.

One clear and sustained hemodynamic effect of somatostatin analogues in patients with cirrhosis is certainly the ability to prevent postprandial splanchnic hyperemia. Octreotide prevents HVPG, ABF and hepatic blood flow increases in response to food intake [19–21]. Both octreotide and lanreotide have been shown to blunt, for as long as 7 h, meal-induced superior mesenteric arterial and portal blood flow changes [22, 23]. A direct link between meals and the circadian pattern of portal pressure and onset of variceal hemorrhage [24, 25] is difficult to establish. It can be speculated that the ability of somatostatin analogues to prevent postprandial splanchnic hyperemia might have some relevance to the prevention of rebleeding in patients with portal hypertension.

Renal blood flow changes after somatostatin or octreotide administration seem to vary over time. In normal subjects, acute somatostatin infusion is associated with a significant reduction in renal plasma flow, glomerular filtration rate, free water clearance and urinary volume [26]. In patients with diabetes, similar changes after octreotide infusion were found to correlate to changes in glucagon plasma concentration [27]. In patients with cirrhosis and ascites, acute administration of somatostatin also impaired glomerular filtration and sodium excretion, but this appeared to be unrelated to neurohumoral changes [28]. However, undesired renal effects of octreotide seem to be no longer detectable after 15 days of bidaily subcutaneous administration, suggesting that, alike other hemodynamic effects, renal hemodynamic changes may be transient [29]. In addition, long-term administration of octreotide in fact had a favorable effect on sodium retention in rats rendered cirrhotic by carbon tetrachloride [30]. Thus, although both somtostatin and octreotide have unfavorable immediate renal hemodynamic effects, it is probable that undesired renal vasoconstriction does not persist over time.

In summary, splanchnic, alike systemic hemodynamic changes after somatostatin or octreotide, appear to be short-lived and subject to rapid desensitization, providing the rationale for bolus infusion, perhaps in a repeated manner, in patients with variceal hemorrhage. In the case of somatostatin, this may be associated with a rebound phenomenon. It has been suggested that increasing the dose of somatostatin might overcome some of these limitations and increase the efficacy of the drug to control acute variceal bleeding [13, 31]. Finally, it should be stressed that somatostatin or its derivatives, in contrast with terlipressin, do not induce clear-cut changes in variceal pressure and that the mechanism of acute hemodynamic effects induced by these drugs remains largely unknown.

Side Effects of Somatostatin or Octreotide

Possible adverse effects of any pharmacological therapy have major strategic implications in patients with acute variceal bleeding [32]. First, these patients are frequently in an unstable hemodynamic condition and may have severe underlying liver disease, that should not be further deteriorated by inappropriate drug use. Second, drugs, in contrast with interventional endoscopy, represent the only immediate therapy that can be administered before hemodynamic stabilization, before transfer to a specialized center, sometimes even before arrival at hospital [33]. Third, physicians in charge of these patients often act under the pressure of emergency and do not have access to a complete medical history, which renders sometimes hazardous the recognition of coronary heart disease or peripheral arterial insufficiency.

Somatostatin, in short-term use, has not been responsible for severe adverse effects and has an excellent safety profile. Rapid injection may be followed by abdominal pain, diarrhea and hot flushes, usually of minimal intensity, which did not necessitate termination of therapy in the studies involving patients with cirrhosis. In a meta-analysis of trials with somatostatin in patients with acute variceal bleeding, the median complication rate was 6.5% [34], making somatostatin the safest therapy available in this setting. Octreotide short-term use can induce flushes, abdominal pain and nausea, very similar in incidence rate and intensity to what is observed after somatostatin.

Both somatostatin and octreotide acute administration are followed by a transient and moderate elevation in pulmonary arterial pressure [11, 12]. Although more than 2% of patients with cirrhosis have elevated baseline pulmonary arterial pressures [35], this effect of somatostatin and its derivatives has not been reported to be associated with detectable clinical events. However, one patient has been reported to suffer from pulmonary edema while receiving octreotide for variceal hemorrhage [36]. An isolated case of octreotide liver toxicity has been reported [37], possibly due to liver ischemia in relation to a decrease in liver blood flow. Isolated cases of paralytic ileus have also been reported, which resolved after cessation of octreotide administration [36, 38]. Mild hypoglycemia, followed by a rise in serum glucose, has been described in normal subjects, both after somatostatin or octreotide infusion [39]. In patients with acute variceal bleeding, two studies [36, 38] reported a higher number of patients with hyperglycemia in the group treated by octreotide compared to the placebo group.

An incidence of 20–30% of gallstones has been reported in patients with acromegaly after long-term use of octreotide. In patients with cirrhosis, who frequently have pigment gallstones in relation chronic liver disease, this would represent a concern if somatostatin derivatives were to be administered for long periods of time.

Somatostatin versus Placebo in Acute Variceal Bleeding (table 1)

Only three randomized controlled trials have compared somatostatin to placebo in the control of variceal hemorrhage. In the first study, Valenzuela et al. [40] administered somatostatin, 250 µg bolus, followed by 250 µg/h continuous infusion for 30 h. The bolus was repeated if the bleeding was not controlled. Somatostatin had no efficacy on bleeding control in these patients. No difference in the mortality at 6 weeks was observed. The main limitation of this multicenter study is that, out of 102 patients included, 18 were excluded in retrospect from final analysis. The second study [41] was the only one to show some efficacy of somatostatin over placebo. It has been commented that the rate of spontaneous cessation of bleeding (41%) was unusually low in this study. Finally, a third study from Copenhagen [42] had the major limitation of an extended inclusion period (5 years for 86 patients). A meta-analysis of the three studies by the same authors [42] emphasized the differences in doses, durations of treatment and average numbers of units transfused in the three studies and failed to evidence any significant efficacy of somatostatin compared to placebo.

There has been no published controlled trial comparing octreotide to placebo in acute variceal bleeding.

Somatostatin or Octreotide versus Endoscopic Therapy (table 2)

Four RCTs compared somatostatin to sclerotherapy in patients with variceal bleeding [43–46]. The success rate of somatostatin or sclerotherapy for bleeding control was similar in three of these studies; in the fourth one [43], only published in abstract form, the success rate was lower in the somatostatin group. Although all four studies report a higher complication rate in patients receiving sclerotherapy, only two [45, 46] discriminated 'major complications' which were also more frequent in the group treated with sclerotherapy. The largest of these four trials [46] extended these findings to the 6-week risk of rebleeding which did not differ between the two groups (14 vs. 15%).

Four trials, two or which only published in abstract form, compared octreotide to sclerotherapy [36, 47–49]. None of these studies showed a significant difference in bleeding control or mortality between groups. It is important to emphasize that in the two largest studies [36, 47], patients randomized to the octreotide group also received sclerotherapy as soon as possible after the 48-hour study period. The largest trial [36] concluded that octreotide appeared to be as effective as injection sclerotherapy in the control of acute variceal bleeding. However, because late mortality due to multiorgan failure was more frequent in the octreotide group, the authors also expressed concerns about the safety of this treatment. The other fully published study [47] was criticized for insufficient statistical power [50].

Table 1. Somatostatin versus placebo in acute variceal bleeding

Drug used	Study	Total number of patients	Dose	Duration	Control of bleeding		Mortality (6 weeks)	
					drug	placebo	drug	placebo
Somatostatin	Valenzuela, 1989 [40]	84	250 μg bolus + 250 μg/h infusion	30 h	65%	83%	31%	25%
	Burroughs, 1990 [41]	120	250 μg infusion	5 days	64%[a]	41%	16%	12%
	Gotzsche, 1995 [42]	86	250 μg infusion	24 h	62%	70%	38%	36%

[a] $p = 0.0545$ compared to placebo group.

Table 2. Somatostatin or octreotide compared to endoscopic sclerotherapy

Drug used	Study	Total number of patients	Dose	Duration	Control of bleeding[a]		Complication rate		Mortality[b]	
					drug	sclerotherapy	drug	sclerotherapy	drug	sclerotherapy
Somatostatin	Di Febo, 1990 [43]	47	250 μg/h infusion	48 h	92%	89%	8%	4%	26%	21%
	Shields, 1992 [44]	80	250 μg bolus each day + 250 μg/h infusion	5 days	77%	83%	13%	29%	31%	30%
	Planas, 1994 [45]	70	250 μg/h infusion	5 days	60%	68%	14%	29[c]	28%	23%
	Escorsell, 1998 [46]	169	250 μg boluses: initial + every 24 h + 250 μg/h infusion	5 days	15%[d] 14%[e]	15%[d] 15%[e]	4%	24%[c]	9%[e]	9%[e]
Octreotide	Sung, 1993 [47]	98	50 μg bolus + 50 μg/h infusion	48 h	84%	90%	10%	37%	20%	27%
	Kravetz, 1996 [48]	45	100 μg bolus, initial + 50 μg/h infusion, 48 h + 100 μg TID SC, 72 h	5 days	88%	92%	36%	32%	20%	8%
	Poo, 1996 [49]	43	50 μg/h infusion	48 h	95%	90%	5%	5%	14%	25%
	Jenkins, 1997 [36]	150	50 μg/h infusion	48 h	85%	82%	19%	26%[f]	31%	17%

[a] At 48 h, unless mentioned otherwise.
[b] Mortality at 30 days, unless mentioned otherwise.
[c] $p < 0.05$, compared to somatostatin.
[d] Rebleeding at 120 h.
[e] At 42 days.
[f] Severe complications: 2 in the octreotide group, 1 in the sclerotherapy group.

A meta-analytic review of these studies was published in 1995 [51] in which the short-term efficacy of somatostatin or octreotide appeard to be comparable to that of sclerotherapy. It has been suggested that, since these trials were usually conducted in referral centers, optimal chances had been given to endoscopic therapy, which is not always the case in everyday life. The complication rate was significantly higher in patients treated by sclerotherapy, but it should be noted that, except in one study [45], most reported complications were mild. Finally, somatostatin or octreotide, which have been used for a short period in most of these studies, by no means represented definitive therapy in these patients, the majority of whom also received endoscopic therapy after 48 h. Thus, somatostatin appears as a viable first-line treatment to control acute variceal bleeding, probably the safest alternative to emergency endoscopic therapy.

The data on octreotide compared to emergency sclerotherapy is more heterogeneous than that published on similar use of somatostatin, mainly because the published trials were small and used different doses and administration schedules. In addition, in the only study involving

Table 3. Endoscopic therapy alone or associated with octreotide

Drug used	Study (type of endoscopic therapy)	Total number of patients	Dose	Duration	Rebleeding rate 5 days/30 days		Complication rate		Mortality	
					endoscopic therapy alone	combination	endoscopic therapy alone	combination	endoscopic therapy alone	combination
Octreotide	Sung, 1995 [52] (ligation)	94	50 μg bolus + 50 μg/h infusion	5 days	38%/38%	8%/8%[a]	NR	NR	23%[b]	11%[b]
	Besson, 1995 [38] (sclerotherapy)	199	25 μg/h infusion	5 days	29%/34%	13%[a]/20%	39%	33%	12%[c]	12%[c]

[a] $p<0.05$ compared to endoscopic therapy alone.
[b] Mortality at 30 days.
[c] Mortality at 15 days.

more than 50 patients per group [36], although overall differences in efficacy or mortality did not reach statistical significance, the number of patients dying from late-onset multiorgan failure was significantly higher in the octreotide group. This has not been explained by the authors or by previous studies. Accepting a type II error of < 10%, a sample size of 140 patients is needed to have a 90% chance to detect a 20% difference between two treatments. Thus, none of these studies had the statistical power to detect small differences in efficacy or survival. Further studies are needed before octreotide can be recommended as a safe alternative for emergency sclerotherapy or ligation.

Another endoscopic technique, variceal ligation, was proven to have some superiority over sclerotherapy for long-term prevention of variceal rebleeding. However, the applicability, safety and results of this newer technique in the emergency setting are still debated and have not been compared to that of somatostatin or octreotide.

Endoscopic Therapy plus Somatostatin or Octreotide versus Endoscopic Therapy Alone (table 3)

Three prospective randomized studies compared endoscopic therapy alone to its combination with octreotide. In the first trial [52], variceal ligation alone was compared to the combination of ligation with octreotide infusion, 50 μg bolus, followed by 50 μg/h infusion for 5 days, starting during endoscopy. All patients had repeat ligation at day 5. Unfortunately, there was no placebo and this was an unblinded study. Although no difference was evidenced in the immediate control of bleeding, which was obtained in >90% of the patients in both groups, 18 patients had recurrent variceal bleeding in the group receiving variceal ligation alone, compared to 4 in the group receiving combined therapy ($p<0.05$). Surprisingly, all rebleedings were observed within 48 h of inclusion. This was not associated with a difference in survival between groups. Side effects are not reported in this work.

In the second of these studies, Besson et al. [38] compared sclerotherapy plus placebo to a combination of sclerotherapy and octreotide, 25 μg/h infusion for 5 days, starting immediately after sclerotherapy. This was a double-blind study. Unfortunately, there was an imbalance between groups, with higher Pugh's scores in the placebo group. At day 5, more patients survived without rebleeding in the combination group (87 vs. 71%, $p=0.009$). This difference remained significant after adjustment for Child-Pugh's class and other variables. Consistent with this finding, the number of blood units transfused was lower in the combination group. No difference in mortality at 15 days was evidenced.

Another large multicenter trial, only published in abstract form [53], will also be discussed as an atempt to initiate early pharmacological therapy (see below and table 4), since octreotide or placebo were initiated before sclerotherapy. One hundred and ninety-three patients were randomized to receive octreotide, 50 μg/h infusion for 5 days, or placebo. Mean time from overt bleeding to admission was 3 h, from admission to pharmacotherapy, 3 h, and from pharmacotherapy to endoscopy, 5 h. Sclerotherapy was used at endoscopy when bleeding persisted. No difference between groups was observed in the need to proceed to sclerotherapy, early rebleeding or mortality.

A small additional study [54] compared sclerotherapy alone to the combination of sclerotherapy with somatostatin or octreotide. Although this was not a randomized

Table 4. Early administration of somatostatin or octreotide versus placebo followed by endoscopic sclerotherapy

Drug used	Study	Total number of patients	Dose	Duration	Failure rate (5 days)		Complication rate		Mortality (5 days[a]/42 days)	
					sclero-therapy	combina-tion	sclero-therapy	combina-tion	sclero-therapy	combina-tion
Somastostatin	Avgerinos, 1997 [56]	205	250 μg boluses: initial + if clinical signs of bleeding + before sclerotherapy + 250 μg/h infusion	5 days	55%	35%	37%	36%	18%/27%	9%[b]/23%
Octreotide	Burroughs, 1996 [53]	193	50 μg/h infusion	5 days	69%	64%	NR[c]	NR	NR/27%	NR/22%

a Death or rescue therapy within 120 h.
b $p < 0.05$ compared to sclerotherapy alone.
c NR: not reported.

controlled study and the groups were small, this study also suggested that both somatostatin and octreotide increased the efficacy of sclerotherapy on bleeding control.

Thus, because both fully published studies [38, 52] have been criticized, one because of an imbalance between groups for severity of liver disease, the other for being unblinded, and because the third large study, still unpublished, gave negative results, available data is insufficient to draw the conclusion that combination of octreotide to endoscopic therapy improves bleeding control.

The Case for Early Administration of Pharmacotherapy (table 4)

Levacher et al. [33] conducted the first randomized trial to test potential benefit from pharmacotherapy, administered even before the patients reached the hospital. The rationale for such an early administration derives from evidence linking early hemodynamic events in patients with variceal bleeding and subsequent deterioration of liver function, which is the main cause of death in these patients. These hemodynamic events probably include changes in splanchnic, portocollateral and intrahepatic resistances, as well as the possibility of liver ischemia in response to the presence of blood in the gut, blood transfusion, and systemic hypotension. The pharmacological treatment used in this study [33] was a combination of terlipressin and nitroglycerin. Improved control of the bleeding in the group treated by this combination was associated to a significant reduction in mortality at day 15. Although this study has been criticized for insufficient data on mortality [55], it opened a new concept in the management of patients with cirrhosis and upper gastrointestinal bleeding. Obviously, immediate management by a specialized team and access to endoscopy is rarely offered, and the number of hours elapsed before endoscopic therapy can be performed may be critical.

The European ABOVE study [65] included 205 patients with cirrhosis and upper gastrointestinal bleeding, 152 of whom had variceal bleeding. Immediately after admission, patients were randomized to receive somatostatin, 250 μg boluses (initial, repeated before sclerotherapy, and up to 8 times if clinical signs of bleeding occurred) followed by 250 μg/h infusion for 5 days, or placebo. Sclerotherapy was performed within 8 h of randomization. At the time of emergency endoscopy, less patients had active variceal bleeding in the somatostatin group, compared to the placebo group (35 vs. 56%, $p = 0.012$). Sclerotherapy was significantly easier to perform in the somatostatin group. Death or rescue therapy was less frequent in the somatostatin group, compared to the placebo group (35 vs. 55%, $p = 0.004$). Consistent with the difference in rebleeding rate, the amount of blood transfused was lower in the somatostatin than in the placebo group. There was no difference in adverse effects or mortality between groups.

The international trial coordinated by Burroughs et al. [53] can also be seen as an attempt to evaluate the efficacy of octreotide early administration. Three hours in mean after hospital admission, 193 patients with bleeding esophageal varices were randomized to receive octreotide, 50 μg/h for 5 days or placebo. No boluses were given. Endoscopy was performed a mean of 8 h after admission. Thus the delay between the start of therapy and endoscopy can be calculated to have averaged only 5 h. Sclerotherapy was used for persistent spurting or oozing at endoscopy. No difference was

Table 5. Strategies for the prevention of rebleeding in cirrhosis

Drug used	Study	Number of patients	Dose	Duration	Rebleeding		Complication rate		Mortality	
					octreotide + standard management (15 days/ 42 days)	placebo + standard management (15 days/ 42 days)	octreotide + standard management	placebo + standard management	octreotide + standard management (42 days)	placebo + standard management (42 days)
Octreotide	Primignani, 1995 [57]	58	100 µg 3 times daily s.c.	30 days	31%/NR[a]	34%/NR	NR	NR	38%	22%
	D'Amico, 1998 [58]	262	100 µg 3 times daily s.c.	15 days	24%/37%	28%/46%	3%	1%	20%	15%
		198 eligible to β-blockers of sclerotherapy[b]			15%[c]/28%[c]	27%/42%			10%	8%
		64 not eligible to β-blockers or sclerotherapy[b]			49%/68%	33%/63%			47%	47%
					Rebleeding		Complication rate		Mortality	
					soctreotide + sclerotherapy (6 months)	sclerotherapy alone (6 months)	octreotide + sclerotherapy	sclerotherapy alone	octreotide + sclerotherapy (6 months)	sclerotherapy alone (6 months)
	Jenkins, 1997 [36]	32	50 µg twice daily s.c.	6 months	5%[c]	36%	50% (minor except one)	NR	0%	26%

[a] NR: not reported.
[b] See text.
[c] $p<0.05$ compared to the group without somatostatin or octreotide.

found between the two groups in the need to proceed to sclerotherapy. Since this study is only published in abstract form, it is difficult to know whether or not this 5-hour delay was balanced between groups and allowed the conclusion that early pharmacological therapy failed to control bleeding.

Thus, although the large European ABOVE study [56] is very consistent with an efficacy of early administration of somatostatin on early bleeding and rebleeding control, at this time no such conclusion can be drawn on the efficacy of early octreotide administration.

Octreotide in the Long-Term Prevention of Rebleeding (table 5)

Three studies evaluated extended use of octreotide with the primary end-point of preventing rebleeding. In the first study, Primignani et al. [57] randomized 58 patients, 24 h after variceal bleeding had stopped to receive 100 µg of octreotide subcutaneously 3 times a day, or an identical placebo, up to day 29. Eight of 26 (31%) patients in the combination group rebled, compared with 11 of 32 (34%) in the sclerotherapy group. No difference in complications or mortality was noted.

In a second study, D'Amico et al. [58] compared octreotide to placebo, combined with pragmatic therapy, for the prevention of rebleeding in 262 patients with cirrhosis and upper digestive bleeding. The source of the index bleed was esophageal varices in only 63% of these patients. When the bleeding was controlled (24 h in mean after admission) the patients were randomized to receive octreotide, 100 µg subcutaneously 3 times a day, or placebo starting 52 h in mean from admission during 15 days. This was a double-blind pragmatic trial in which patients also received sclerotherapy and/or β-blockers whenever indicated. Although 15-day cumulative proportions of patients with rebleeding did not differ between the two groups, analysis of the subgroup of patients eligible to sclerotherapy and/or β-blockers showed a significant reduction of rebleeding episodes (35 vs. 18, $p=0.03$), blood transfusions (75 vs. 50, $p=0.04$), and days of stay in hospital (1,544 vs. 1,190, $p=0.0001$) in the octreotide group, compared to the placebo group. The multivariate analysis using a Cox model showed that in this subgroup of patients, and not in the whole group, blood urea nitrogen and octreotide were the only significant predictors of rebleeding. As noted by the authors, statistical flaws in this study relate to posthoc analysis, with insufficient power to reach a p value <0.025 for repeat comparisons.

Finally, Jenkins et al. [59] randomized 32 patients with cirrhosis to receive octreotide, 50 μg twice daily for 6 months in combination to sclerotherapy or sclerotherapy alone. The cause of cirrhosis was dominantly alcoholic and the patients were included 3 weeks after an index variceal bleed. In addition, hepatic vein pressure measurements were recorded at entry and at 6 months. Recurrent variceal bleeding occurred within 6 months in 1 of 16 patients who received combination therapy, versus 7 of 16 who received sclerotherapy alone ($p=0.037$). Even more surprisingly, liver function significantly improved, and wedged hepatic venous pressure decreased at 6 months in the combination group, compared to the sclerotherapy group [60]. Because of insufficient statistical power and lack of information on alcohol abstinence or the causes of death, this unblinded study has been criticized [60].

Concluding comments

From the evidence reviewed in this paper, it appears that somatostatin infusion can be as effective as sclerotherapy in the initial control of bleeding esophageal varices in patients with cirrhosis and is associated with fewer complications. Although this should be confirmed, a large recent trial suggested that somatostatin compared favorably to sclerotherapy, with similar efficacy on 6 week-rebleeding risk and fewer complications [46]. Octreotide also seems to be as effective as endoscopic therapy in the control of acute variceal bleeding. However, the single large trial which compared octreotide to sclerotherapy in patients with acute variceal hemorrhage raised concerns about the safety of this pharmacological therapy in patients with cirrhosis and upper gastrointestinal hemorrhage, in part because late mortality due to multiorgan failure was higher in the octreotide group [36].

The combination of somatostatin or long-acting analogues to endoscopic therapy seems to be one of the most promising approaches in these patients. Early somatostatin infusion with repeat bolus administration, several hours before sclerotherapy is eventually combined, eases the endoscopic procedure and reduces bleeding control failure rate [56]. Undoubtedly, the demonstration that early pharmacological therapy, which requires no specific technical skills, is safe, effective, and can allow optimized elective endoscopic therapy a few hours later, represents a major step in the history of emergency care in patients with cirrhosis and upper intestinal bleeding. Two studies also suggested that octreotide, when combined to sclerotherapy or variceal banding respectively, improves bleeding control. Because these trials raised a number of questions, a conclusion on octreotide use in this setting is premature and more studies should be performed in groups large enough to allow sufficient statistical power.

Recent data suggested that doses of somatostatin larger than those usually recommended may increase its efficacy [31]. Similarly, the question of the most appropriate octreotide dose for future studies remains unsettled. The question of the most efficient doses and administration schedules of somatostatin and its derivatives should be further explored.

Beyond immediate control of the acute bleeding episode, long-term prevention of rebleeding remains an important concern. Recent studies, still to be confirmed, suggest that octreotide combination to β-blockers or sclerotherapy may represent a promising approach in these patients.

Acknowledgment

Immense thanks are due to Ms. Françoise Delacrétaz for expert secretarial help.

References

1 Navarro VJ, Garcia-Tsao G: Variceal hemorrhage. Gastrointest Emerg 1995;11:391–413.

2 Pagliaro L, D'Amico G, Pasta L, Politi F, Vizzini G, Traina S, et al: Portal hypertension in cirrhosis: Natural history; in Bosch J, Groszmann RJ (eds): Portal Hypertension. Pathophysiology and Treatment. Oxford, Blackwell, 1994, pp 72–92.

3 Imperiale TF, Teran JC, McCullough AJ: A meta-analysis of somatostatin versus vasopressin in the management of acute esophageal variceal hemorrhage. Gastroenterology 1995;109:1289–1294.

4 Walker S, Kreichgauer HP, Bode JC: Terlipressin (glypressin) versus somatostatin in the treatment of bleeding esophageal varices – Final report of a placebo-controlled, double-blind study. Z Gastroenterol 1996;34:692–698.

5 Feu F, Ruiz del Arbol L, Banares R, Planas R, Bosch J: Double-blind randomized controlled trial comparing terlipressin and somatostatin for acute variceal hemorrhage. Variceal Bleeding Study Group. Gastroenterology 1996;111:1291–1299.

6 Pedretti G, Elia G, Calzetti C, Magnani GM, Fiaccadori F: Octreotide versus terlipressin in acute variceal hemorrhage in liver cirrhosis. Emergency control and prevention of early rebleeding. Clin Invest 1994;72:653–659.

7 Silvain C, Carpentier S, Sautereau D, Czernichow B, Metreau JM, Fort E, Ingrand P, Boyer J, Pillegand B, Doffel M, et al: Terlipressin plus transdermal nitroglycerin vs octreotide in the control of acute bleeding from esophageal varices: A multicenter randomized trial. Hepatology 1993;18:61–65.
8 De Franchis R: Developing consensus in portal hypertension. J Hepatol 1996;25:390–394.
9 Jenkins SA, Nott DM, Baxter JN: Pharmacokinetics of octreotide in patients with cirrhosis and portal hypertension: Relationship between the plasma levels of the analogue and the magnitude and duration of the reduction in corrected wedged hepatic venous pressure. HPB Surg 1998;11:13–21.
10 Bosch J, Lebrec D, Jenkins SA: Development of analogues: Successes and failures. Scand J Gastroenterol 1998;33(suppl 226):3–13.
11 Gaudin C, Moreau R, Champigneulle B, Soubrane O, Kleber G, Lebrec D: Short-term cardiovascular effects of somatostatin in patients with cirrhosis. Liver 1995;15:236–241.
12 McCormick PA, Chin J, Greeslade L, Karatapanis S, Dick R, Mclntyre N, et al: Cardiovascular effects of octreotide in patients with hepatic cirrhosis. Hepatology 1995;21:1255–1260.
13 Cirera I, Feu F, Luca A, Garcia-Pagan JC, Fernandez M, Escorsell A, Bosch J, Rodes J: Effects of bolus injections and continuous infusions of somatostatin and placebo in patients with cirrhosis: A double-blind hemodynamic investigation. Hepatology 1995;22:106–111.
14 Nishida H, Giostra E, Spahr L, Mentha G, Mitamura K, Hadengue A: Acute effects of somatostatin, octreotide or placebo in patients with cirhosis. A double-blind study. Hepatology 1998;28:235A.
15 Kleber G, Sauerbruch T, Fischer G, Paumgartner G: Somatostatin does not reduce oesophageal variceal pressure in liver cirrhotics. Gut 1988;29:153–156.
16 Nevens F, Van Steenbergen W, Yap SH, Fevery J: Assessment of variceal pressure by continuous non-invasive endoscopic registration: A placebo-controlled evaluation of the effect of terlipressin and octreotide. Gut 1996;38:129–134.
17 Primignani M, Vazzoler MC, Carpinelli L, Nolte A, Hall de Lima MC, Arcidiacono PG: Short-term effect of octreotide on intraoesophageal pressure: A double-blind placebo-controlled study. Eur J Gastroenterol Hepatol 1994;6:1027–1031.
18 Barrioz T, Borderie C, Strock P, Ingrand P, Fort E, Silvain C, Beauchant M: Effects of octreotide on lower esophageal sphincter in patients with cirrhosis and portal hypertension. Dig Dis Sci 1998;43:1566–1571.
19 McCormick PA, Biagini MR, Dick R, Greenslade L, Chin J, Cardin F, Wagstaff D, Mclntyre N, Burroughs AK: Octreotide inhibits the meal-induced increases in the portal venous pressure of cirrhotic patients with portal hypertension: A double-blind, placebo-controlled study. Hepatology 1992;16:1180–1186.
20 Albillos A, Rossi I, Iborra J, Lledo JL, Calleja JL, Barrios C, Garcia P, Escartin P: Octreotide prevents postprandial splanchnic hyperemia in patients with portal hypertension. J Hepatol 1994;21:88–94.
21 Lin HC, Tsai YT, Huang CC, Meng HC, Lee FY, Wang SS, Lee SD, Lo KJ: Effects of octreotide on postprandial systemic and hepatic hemodynamics in patients with postnecrotic cirrhosis. J Hepatol 1994;21:424–429.
22 Buonamico P, Sabba C, Garcia-Tsao G, Berardi E, Antonica G, Ferraioli G, Jensen JE, Lerner E, Taylors KJW, Albano O, Grozmann RJ: Octreotide blunts postprandial splanchnic hyperemia in cirrhotic patients: A double-blind randomized echo-Doppler study. Hepatology 1995; 21:134–139.
23 Mottet C, Sieber CC, Nauer A, Drewe J, Fried R, Larsen F, Beglinger C: Hemodynamic effects of the somatostatin analog lanreotide in humans: Placebo-controlled, cross-over dose-ranging echo-Doppler study. Hepalogy 1998;27:920–925.
24 Garcia-Pagan JC, Feu F, Castells A, Luca A, Hermida RC, Rivera F, Bosch J, Rodes J: Circadian variations of portal pressure and variceal hemorrhage in patients with cirrhosis. Hepatology 1994;19:595–601.
25 Merican I, Sprengers D, McCormick PA, Minoli G, Mclntyre N, Burroughs AK: Diurnal pattern of variceal bleeding in cirrhotic patient. J Hepatol 1993;19:15–22.
26 Vora JP, Owens DR, Ryder R, Atiea J, Luzio S, Hayes TM: Effect of somatostatin on renal function. Br Med J 1986;292:1701–1702.
27 Pedersen MM, Christensen SE, Christiansen JS, Pedersen EB, Mogensen CE, Orskov H: Acute effects of a somatostatin analogue on kidney function in type 1 diabetic patients. Diabet Med 1990;7:304–309.
28 Gines A, Salmeron JM, Gines P, Jimenez W, Salo J, Piera C, Claria J, Rivera F, Arroyo V, Rodes J: Effects of somatostatin on renal function in cirrhosis. Gastroenterology 1992;103: 1868–1874.
29 Malesci A, Tacconi M, Valentini A, Basilico M, Lorenzano E, Salerno F: Octreotide long-term treatment in patients with portal hypertension: Persistent inhibition of postprandial glucagon response without major changes in renal function. J Hepatol 1997;26:816–825.
30 Wang SS, Lee FY, Wu SL, Hwu CM, Chien CH, Lee SD, Tsai YT, Chao Y, Chen CC, Wang PS: Effects of long-term administration of octreotide on sodium retention and atrial natriuretic peptide in carbon tetrachloride-induced cirrhotic rats. J Hepatol 1997;26:1128–1134.
31 Variceal Bleeding Study Group: A multicenter randomized controlled trial comparing different schedules of somatostatin administration in the treatment of acute variceal bleeding. Hepatology 1998;28:770A.
32 Burroughs AK, Planas R, Svoboda P: Optimizing emergency care of upper gastrointestinal bleeding in patients with cirrhosis. Scand J Gastroenterol 1998;33(supple 226):14–24.
33 Levacher S, Letoumelin P, Pateron D, Blaise M, Lapandry C, Pourriat JL: Early administration of terlipressin plus glyceryl trinitrate to control active upper gastrointestinal bleeding in cirrhotic patients. Lancet 1995;346:865–868.
34 D'Amico G, Pagliaro L, Bosch J: The treatment of portal hypertension: A meta-analytic review. Hepatology 1995;22:332–354.
35 Hadengue A, Benhayoun MK, Lebrec D, Benhamou JP: Pulmonary hypertension complicating portal hypertension: Prevalence and relation to splanchnic hemodynamics. Gastroenterology 1991;100:520–528.
36 Jenkins SA, Shields R, Davies M, Elias E, Turnbull AJ, Bassendine MF, James OF, Iredale JP, Vyas SK, Arthur MJ, Kingsnorth AN, Sutton R: A multicentre randomised trial comparing octreotide and injection sclerotherapy in the management and outcome of acute variceal haemorrhage. Gut 1997;41:526–533.
37 Minocha A, Dean HA Jr: Octreotide-induced acute hepatic toxicity. Am J Gastroenterol 1991; 81:525–526.
38 Besson I, Ingrand P, Person B, Boutroux D, Heresbach D, Bernard P, et al: Sclerotherapy with or without octreotide for acute variceal bleeding. N Engl J Med 1995;333:555–560.
39 Sherwin RS, Hendler R, DeFronzo R, Wahren J, Felic P: Glucose homeostasis during prolonged suppression of glucagon and insulin secretion by somatostatin. Proc Natl Acad Sci USA 1977; 74:348–352.
40 Valenzuela JE, Shubert T, Fogel RM, Strong RM, Levine J, Mills RR, et al: A multicenter, randomized, double-blind trial of somatostatin in the management of acute esophageal varices. Hepatology 1989;10:958–961.
41 Burroughs AK, McCormick PA, Hughes MD, Sprengers S, D'Heygere F, Mclntyre N: Randomized, double-blind, placebo-controlled trial of somatostatin for variceal bleeding. Gastroenterology 1990;99:1388–1395.
42 Gotzsche PC, Gjorup I, Bonnen H, Brahe NEB, Becker U, Burcharth F: Somatostatin versus placebo in bleeding oesophageal varices: Randomized trial and meta-analysis. BMJ 1995;310: 1495–1498.
43 Di Febo C, Siringo M, Vacirca M, Santoro P, Merighi S, Mustafa A, et al: Somatostatin (SMS) and urgent sclerotherapy in active oesophageal variceal bleeding (abstract). Gastroenterology 1990;98:583.
44 Shields R, Jenkins SA, Baxter JN, Kingsnorth AN, Ellenbogen S, Makin CA, et al: A prospective randomized controlled trial comparing the efficacy of somatostatin with injection sclerotherapy in the control of oesophageal varices. J Hepatol 1992;16:128–137.
45 Planas R, Quer JC, Boix J, Canet J, Armengol M, Cabre E, et al: A prospective randomized trial comparing somatostatin and sclerotherapy in the treatment of acute variceal bleeding. Hepatology 1994;20:370–375.

46 Escorsell A, Bordas JM, del Arbol LE, Jaramillo JL, Planas R, Banares R, Albillos A, Bosch J: Randomized controlled trial of sclerotherapy versus somatostatin infusion in the prevention of early rebleeding following acute variceal hemorrhage in patients with cirrhosis. Variceal Bleeding Study Group. J Hepatol 1998; 29:779–788.
47 Sung JJ, Sydney Chung SC, Lai CW, Chan FKL, Leung JWC, Yung MY, et al: Octreotide infusion or emergency sclerotherapy for variceal haemorrhage. Lancet 1993;342:1486.
48 Kravetz D and Group for the Study of Portal Hypertension: Octreotide versus sclerotherapy in the treatment of acute variceal bleeding. Prospective clinical controlled trial. Hepatology 1996;24:206A.
49 Poo JL, Bosques F, Garduno R, Marin E, Moran MA, Bobadilla J, Maldonado EP, Morales D, Garcia-Cantu D, Uribe M: Octreotide versus emergency sclerotherapy in acute variceal hemorrhage in liver cirrhosis. A randomized multicenter study. Gastroenterology 1996;110: A1297.
50 Altman DG: Octreotide infusion versus injection sclerotherapy. Lancet 1993;342:1486.
51 Avgerinos A, Armonis A, Raptis S: Somatostatin or octreotide versus endoscopic therapy in acute variceal hemorrhage: A meta-analysis study. J Hepatol 1995;110:247–248.
52 Sung JJ, Chung SC, Yung MY, Lai CW, Lau JY, Lee YT, et al: Prospective randomized study of effect of octreotide on rebleeding from oesophageal varices after endoscopic ligation. Lancet 1995;346:1666–1669.
53 Burroughs AK and the International Octreotide Varices Study Group: Double-blind RCT of 5 days octreotide versus placebo, associated with sclerotherapy for trial failures. Hepatology 1996;24(suppl 4):352A.
54 Signorelli S, Negrini F, Paris B, Bonelli M, Girola M: Sclerotherapy with or without octreotide in the treatment of acute variceal haemorrhage: Our experience (abstract). Gastroenterology 1996;110:A1326.
55 Burroughs AK, Patch D: Therapeutic benefit of vasoactive drugs for acute variceal bleeding: A real pharmacological effect or a side-effect, or definition in trials? Hepatology Elsewhere 1996;24:737–739.
56 Avgerinos A, Nevens F, Raptis S, Fevery J, and the ABOVE Study Group: Early administration of somatostatin and efficacy of sclerotherapy in acute oesophageal variceal bleeds: The European Acute Bleeding Oesophageal Variceal Episodes (ABOVE) Randomized Trial. Lancet 1997;350:1495–1499.
57 Primignani M, Andreoni B, Carpinelli L, Capria A, Rocchi G, Lorenuzini I, et al: Sclerotherapy plus octreotide versus sclerotherapy alone in the prevention of early rebleeding from oesophageal varices: A randomized, double-blind, placebo-controlled, multicenter trial. New Italian Endoscopic Club. Hepatology 1995;21: 1322–1327.
58 D'Amico G, Politi AF, Morabito A, D'Antoni A, Guerrera D, Giannuoli G, Traina M, Vizzini G, Pagliaro L and the Liver Study Group of Cervello Hospital: Octreotide compared with placebo in a treatment strategy for early rebleeding in cirrhosis. A double-blind randomized pragmatic trial. Hepatology 1998;28: 1206–1214.
59 Jenkins SA, Baxter JN, Critchley M, Kingsnorth AN, Makin CA, Ellenbogen S, Grime JS, Love JG, Sutton R: Randomised trial of octreotide for long-term management of cirrhosis after variceal haemorrhage. BMJ 1997;315: 1338–1341.
60 Patch D, Burroughs A: Octreotide for cirrhosis after variceal bleeding. Authors' claims for octreotide were not justified. BMJ 1998;316:1607.

Digestion

Digestion 1999;60(suppl 2):42–46

Octreotide in the Treatment of Refractory Diarrhea

M. Fried

Department of Gastroenterology, University Hospital, Zürich, Switzerland

Key Words
Octreotide · AIDS · Chemotherapy · Refractory diarrhea

Abstract
Refractory chronic diarrhea that does not respond to specific antimicrobial therapy or standard unspecific medication may present a challening and serious clinical problem. Octreotide is a candidate drug for the treatment of these patients as it inhibits gastrointestinal motility, pancreatic secretion and inhibits intestinal absorption. Only few mostly uncontrolled studies in small patient groups were published evaluating the efficacy of octreotide in the treatment of patients with chemotherapy-induced diarrhea, short-bowel syndrome, AIDS-associated diarrhea and other conditions with chronic diarrhea not responding to standard treatment. Most of these studies are not conclusive as they yielded either negative or controversial results. Octreotide may be tried in the treatment of refractory diarrhea, in particular AIDS-associated diarrhea if patients do not respond to conventional treatment strategies. Well-designed controlled trials in large patient groups are needed in order to define the place of octreotide in the treatment of patients with refractory diarrhea.

Refractory chronic diarrhea, defined as diarrhea of more than 14 days' duration that does not respond to either specific therapy or to usual antidiarrheal preparations, may constitute a serious and challenging clinical event. Diarrhea occurring in several conditions such as HIV, chemotherapy, in patients with diabetes mellitus and intestinal graft-versus-host disease may fail to respond to conventional treatment applying specific antimicrobial drugs or standard unspecific medications.

The rationale for the use of octreotide in the treatment of refractory diarrhea is based on its effects on multiple locations of the gastrointestinal tract where somatostatin receptors have been identified. Octreotide inhibits gastrointestinal motility, gastric and pancreatic exocrine secretions, the release of several gastrointestinal peptides such as VIP, PMI, 5-HT and splanchnic blood flow and induces net water and electrolyte absorption. All these effects may contribute to the potential antidiarrheal actions of octreotide. Paradoxically some of these actions of octreotide might per se cause diarrhea (e.g. inhibition of pancreatic exocrine secretion), a well-known side effect of therapy with octreotide.

In the following chapters some important potential clinical applications of octreotide are discussed mainly focusing on controlled clinical studies.

AIDS-Associated Diarrhea

Chronic diarrhea in patients with AIDS may significantly contribute to the morbidity and mortality of the disease. Diarrhea may persist in these patients despite treatment with specific antimicrobial drugs and nonspecific antidiarrheal agents.

Seven uncontrolled studies have been published (table 1) demonstrating the efficacy of octreotide to control diarrhea with a response rate between 41 and 100% [1–7]. In a multicenter study, 21 of 51 patients responded

KARGER
Fax +41 61 306 12 34
E-Mail karger@karger.ch
www.karger.ch

0012–2823/99/0608–0042$17.50/0

Accessible online at:
http//BioMedNet.com/karger

M. Fried, MD
University Hospital Zürich – Gastroenterology
Rämistrasse 100, CH–8091 Zurich (Switzerland)
Tel. +41 1 255 8548, Fax +41 1 255 4503
E-Mail gasfrc@usz.unizh.ch

Table 1. AIDS-related diarrhea, uncontrolled studies

Group (first author)	Ref.	n	Response, %
Montaner	1	32	57
Manfredi	2	6	100
Moroni	3	13	69
Romeu	4	25	76
Fanning	5	17	45
Cello	6	1	41
Liberti	7	11	100

Table 2. AIDS-related diarrhea, controlled studies

Group (first author)	Ref.	Single-blind	Double-blind	n	Comparison	Duration, days	Response, %
Compean	8	+		20	Placebo Loperamide Diphenoxylate	10	60 vs. 20
Beaugerie	9			13	Acetorphan (crossover)	14	23 vs. 31
Simon	10		+	129	Placebo	21	48 vs. 39

to a daily dose of 150 μg octreotide for 48 h with a fall of stool frequency and volume [6].

Hitherto three controlled studies (table 2) have been performed evaluating the therapeutic effect of octreotide in AIDS-associated diarrhea [8–10]. In a large multicenter, double-blind, placebo-controlled study in 129 patients, the effect of octreotide was evaluated during a 21-day treatment schedule [10]. The trial included an initial double-blind, placebo-controlled study with an octreotide dose between 300 and 900 μg/day for 4 weeks. This study was followed by an open-label, dose-escalation phase with starting doses of 300 μg/day weekly increasing in 100-μg steps up to a maximum dose of 1,500 μg/day [10]. The response rate to octreotide was 48% as compared to 39% during placebo, which was not significantly different. However, in the open-label phase of the study, octreotide had a significant effect on both stool volume and frequency resulting in a 39% lower stool frequency and 42% lower stool volume at a dose of 1,500 μg/day [10]. This study was criticized for the lack of a control of the patients' compliance, the heterogeneity in the study population and the lack of a standardized patients' diet [11].

The two other controlled studies are of limited value due to problems in their study design. Thus only a small number of patients [8, 9] were included and the studies performed either not blinded [9] or in a single-blinded fashion [8]. In one of these two studies, octreotide (300–1200 μg/day) was given to a patient group and compared to another group of patients treated with loperamide and diphenoxylate [8]. More patients in the octreotide group (6/10) had a positive response as compared to the control group (2/8). In the other study, acetorphan and octreotide (300–1200 μg/day) were given in a crossover fashion to 13 patients [9]. Patients treated with octreotide had a similar response rate (4/13) as those treated with acetorphan (3/13).

In summary, the published data do not equivocally support the use of octreotide in the treatment of AIDS-associated diarrhea. However, none of the published trials has an ideal study design to exclude a possible beneficial role of octreotide in this condition. In future trials more homogenous patient populations should be evaluated prominently including patients with secretory diarrhea with high stool outputs. The diet of the patients should be standardized and the patient's compliance assured. The study duration should be sufficiently long and the effect of high doses of octreotide should be investigated [11].

Chemotherapy-Induced Diarrhea

Chemotherapy may induce diarrhea in up to 20% of cancer patients. It may constitute a severe problem contributing to diminished patient compliance, prolonged hospitalization and may even become live-threatening. Symptomatic treatment with drugs like loperamide and diphenoxylate often fail and peroral medication may be unfeasible.

Four uncontrolled studies were published (table 3) including 16–35 patients treated with 5-fluorouracil [12] alone or in combination with leucovorin [13, 14] and

Table 3. Chemotherapy-induced diarrhea, uncontrolled studies

Group (first author)	Ref.	n	Response, %
Petrelli	13	16	94
Wasserman	15	14	86
Cascinu	14	27	96
Wadler	12	35	74

Table 4. Chemotherapy-induced diarrhea, controlled studies

Group (first author)	Ref.	Single-blind	Double-blind	n	Comparison	Duration, days	Response, %
Cascinu	17	+		41	Loperamide	3	95 vs. 15
Geller	16			36	Loperamide	2	56 vs. 92
Cascinu	18		+[1]	43	Placebo	1	95 vs. 25

[1] Octreotide given *before* cisplatin.

different high-dose chemotherapy regimens including cisplatin [15]. Response rates to octreotide ranged between 74 and 96%.

There are three controlled trials including 36–41 patients (table 4). In two studies octreotide was given after the occurrence of diarrhea and compared to loperamide [16, 17]. In one study, octreotide vs. placebo was given as a prophylactic measure in patients who already developed diarrhea during a previous chemotherapy with cisplatin [18]. Only one study was double-blind [18], one trial was conducted in a single-blind fashion [17], another study was not blinded [10]. The injection of octreotide before chemotherapy resulted in a markedly lower diarrhea frequency (5%) as compared to 75% after placebo. However, in a recent uncontrolled trial no prophylactic effect of octreotide in the prevention of 5-fluorouracil-induced diarrhea was observed [19]. In the two other trials where octreotide was given after the occurrence of diarrhea, opposite results were obtained. In one trial [17] octreotide was more effective than loperamide (95 vs. 15%) whereas in the other trial [16] octreotide was inferior to loperamide (56 vs. 92%).

In summary, only few controlled data are available on the efficiency of octreotide in the treatment of chemotherapy-induced diarrhea presenting contradictory results. Octreotide might have a place in the prophylaxis of diarrhea after chemotherapy, for example with cisplatin. However, there is yet no proven effect of octreotide in the treatment of chemotherapy-induced diarrhea. Further studies in larger patient groups are necessary to clarify the role of octreotide in the treatment of chemotherapy-induced diarrhea.

Short-Bowel Syndrome

Patients with extensive small-bowel resections mostly because of Crohn's disease may suffer from excessive losses of fluid and electrolytes. Some of these patients are difficult to treat by conventional measures and may require parenteral nutrition.

In three uncontrolled studies in a small number of patients, octreotide was only marginally effective in treating diarrhea resulting in a highly variable response rate with a reduction in stool outputs between 16 and 72% [20–22]. In the only placebo-controlled study in 6 patients, octreotide caused a ~50% reduction of stool effluent [23]. The reduction in stool mass can probably be maintained over prolonged time periods of several months [20, 22, 23].

The small number of patients studied and the variable response rates do not allow to judge the clinical value of octreotide in the treatment of patients with short-bowel syndrome. In addition, though octreotide probably reduces intestinal outputs in some of these patients, it is improbable that it would change the treatment by allowing to proceed to oral instead of parenteral nutrition.

Graft-Versus-Host Disease

Diarrhea after bone marrow transplantation as a consequence of acute graft-versus-host disease or drug effects can be severe and may be associated with malnutrition contributing to a high morbidity in these patients.

Treatment with octreotide resulted in a response rate between 50 and 100% in three uncontrolled studies including 6–24 patients [24–27]. In the largest study with an 85% response rate, a high dose of octreotide (1,500 μg/day) was employed [24].

Controlled randomized trials in larger patient groups are required and planned [24] to assess the effectiveness of high doses of octreotide in the management of acute graft-versus-host disease.

Miscellaneous Indications

In patients with dumping syndrome after gastrectomy and vagotomy, octreotide was effective in 6 of 14 patients in an uncontrolled study [28]. In a controlled double-blind study in 16 patients, treatment with octreotide resulted in a clinical benefit in all patients as compared to a 20% placebo response [29].

In three case reports, octreotide was successful in the treatment of severe refractory diarrhea in patients with diabetes mellitus [30–32].

Improvement of diarrhea by the injection of octreotide was described in enteric infections such as cryptosporidiasis [33]. In a controlled study involving 33 patients with diarrhea due to *Vibrio cholerae*, octreotide treatment reduced the duration of diarrhea but not stool volumes [34].

Other applications of octreotide were described in several case reports. Thus octreotide was effective in the treatment of diarrhea after hemicolectomy [35], systemic sclerosis [36], after celiac plexus block [37] and in villous rectal adenoma [38].

Conclusions

Octreotide has been applied in the treatment of refractory diarrhea of different origin. Most of these studies are not conclusive as they yielded either negative or controversial results, were conducted in small patient groups or have other problems in their study design. For the time being, there is no established role for octreotide in the treatment of refractory diarrhea. Octreotide may be employed in the treatment of AIDS-associated diarrhea if patients do not respond to specific treatment of a pathogen and standard therapy of diarrhea. Well-designed controlled trials in large patient groups are needed in order to define the place of octreotide in the treatment of patients with refractory diarrhea.

References

1 Montaner JSG, Harris AG: Octreotide therapy in AIDS-related refractory diarrhea: Results of a multicentre Canadian-European study. AIDS 1995;9:209–210.

2 Manfredi R, Vezzadani P, Fanti MP, Chiodo F: Vasoactive intestinal polypeptide secretion and refractory diarrhea in patients with AIDS or AIDS-related complex. Scand J Infect Dis 1994;26:55–57.

3 Moroni M, Esposito R, Cernuschi M, Franzetti F, Carosi GP, Fiori GP: Treatment of AIDS-related refractory diarrhoea with octreotide. Digestion 1993;54(suppl 1):30–32.

4 Romeu J, Miro JM, Sirera G, Mallolas J, Arnal J, Valls ME, Tortosa F, Clotet B, Foz M: Efficacy of octreotide in the management of chronic diarrhoea in AIDS. AIDS 1991;5:1495–1499.

5 Fanning M, Monte M, Sutherland LR, Froadhead M, Murphy GF, Harris AG: Pilot study of Sandostatin (octreotide) therapy of refractory HIV-associated diarrhea. Dig Dis Sci 1991;36:476–480.

6 Cello JP, Grendell JH, Basuk P, Simon D, Weiss L, Wittner M, Rood RP, Wilcox M, Forsmark CE, Read AE, Satow JA, Weikel CS, Beaumont C: Effect of octreotide on refractory AIDS-associated diarrhea. Ann Int Med 1991;115:705–710.

7 Liberti A, Bisogno A, Izzo E: Octreotide treatment in secretory and cryptosporidial diarrhea in patients with acquired immunodeficiency syndrome: Clinical evaluation. J Chemotherapy 1992;4:303–305.

8 Compean DG, Jimenez JR, Guzman de la Garza F, Saenz C, Maldonado H, Barragan RF, Michel H: Octreotide therapy of large-volume refractory AIDS-associated diarrhea: A randomized controlled trial. AIDS 1994;8:1563–1567.

9 Beaugerie L, Baumer P, Chaussade S, Berard H, Rozenbaum W, Pialoux G, Le Quintrec Y, Schwartz JC, Lecomte JM: Treatment of refractory diarrhea in AIDS with acetorphan and octreotide: Randomized cross-over study. Gastroenterology 1993;104:A664.

10 Simon DM, Cello JP, Valenzuela J, Levy R, Dickerson G, Goodgame R, Brown M, Lyche K, Fessel WJ, Grendel J, Wilcox CM, Afdhal N, Fogel R, Reeves-Darby V, Stern J, Smith O, Graziano F, Pleakow D, Flanigan T, Schubert T, Loveless M, Eron L, Basuk P, Bonacini M, Orenstein J: Multicenter trial of octreotide in patients with refractory acquired immunodeficiency syndrome-associated diarrhea. Gastroenterology 1995;108:1753–1760.

11 Kotler DP: Octreotide therapy for human immunodeficiency virus-associated diarrhea: Pitfalls in drug development. Gastroenterology 1995;108:1939–1941.

12 Wadler S, Haynes H, Wiernik PH: Phase I trial of the somatostatin analog octreotide acetate in the treatment of fluoropyrimidine-induced diarrhea. J Clin Oncol 1995;13:222–226.

13 Petrelli NJ, Rodriguez M, Rustum Y, Herrera L, Creaven P: Bowel rest, intravenous hydration, and continuous high-dose infusion of octreotide acetate for the treatment of chemotherapy-induced diarrhea in patients with colorectal carcinoma. Cancer 1993;72:1543–1546.

14 Cascinu S, Fedeli A, Fedeli SL, Catalano G: Control of chemotherapy-induced diarrhoea with octreotide in patients receiving 5-fluorouracil. Eur J Cancer 1992;28:482–483.

15 Wasserman E, Hidalgo M, Hornedo J, Cortes-Funes H: Octreotide for hematopoietic support-dependent high-dose chemotherapy-related diarrhea: Dose finding study and evaluation of efficacy. Bone Marrow Transplant 1997;20:711–714.

16 Geller RB, Gilmore CE, Dix SP, Lin LS, Topping DL, Davidson TG, Holland HK, Wingard JR: Randomized trial of loperamide versus dose escalation of octreotide acetate for chemotherapy-induced diarrhea in bone marrow transplant and leukemia patients. Am J Hematol 1995;50:167–172.

17 Cascinu S, Fedeli A, Fedeli SL, Catalano G: Octreotide versus loperamide in the treatment of fluorouracil-induced diarrhea: A randomized trial. J Clin Oncol 1993;11:148–151.
18 Cascinu S, Fedeli A, Fedeli SL, Catalano G: Control of chemotherapy-induced diarrhea with octreotide. Oncology 1994;51:70–73.
19 Meropol NJ, Blumenson LE, Creaven PJ: Octreotide does not prevent diarrhea in patients treated with weekly 5-fluorouracil plus high-dose leucovorin. Am J Clin Oncol 1998;2:135–138.
20 Cooper JC, Williams NS, King RFGJ, Barker MCJ: Effects of a long-acting somatostatin analogue in patients with severe ileostomy diarrhoea. Br J Surg 1986;73:128–131.
21 Rodrigues CA, Lennard-Jones JE, Thompson DG, Farthing MJG: The effects of octreotide, soy polysaccharide, codeine and loperamide on nutrient, fluid and electrolyte absorption in the short bowel syndrome. Aliment Pharmacol Ther 1989;3:159–169.
22 Nightingale JMD, Walker ER, Burnham WR, Farthing MJG, Lennard-Jones JE: Octreotide (a somatostatin analogue) improves the quality of life in some patients with a short intestine. Aliment Pharmacol Ther 1989;3:367–373.
23 Ladefoged K, Christensen KC, Hegnohoj J, Jarnum S: Effect of a long-acting somatostatin analogue SMS 201-995 on jejunostomy effluents in patients with severe short bowel syndrome. Gut 1989;30:943–949.
24 Ippoliti C, Champlin R, Bugazia N, Przepiorka D, Neumann J, Giralt S, Khour I, Gajewski J: Use of octreotide in the symptomatic management of diarrhea induced by graft-versus-host disease in patients with hematologic malignancies. J Clin Oncol 1997;11:3350–3354.
25 Morton AJP, Durrant STS: Efficacy of octreotide in controlling refractory diarrhea following bone marrow transplantation. Clin Transplant 1995;9:205–208.
26 Pamela E, Dunitz J, Rogosheske J, Weisdorf D: Use of a somatostatin analogue, octreotide acetate, in the management of acute gastrointestinal graft-versus-host disease. Am J Med 1991; 90:707–710.
27 Crouch MA, Restino MS, Cruz JM, Perry JJ, Hurd DD: Octreotide acetate in refractory bone marrow transplant-associated diarrhea. Ann Pharmacother 1996;30:331–336.
28 Mackie CR, Jenkins SA, Hartley MN: Treatment of severe postvagotomy/postgastrectomy symptoms with the somatostatin analogue octreotide. Br J Surg 1991;78:1338–1343.
29 Geer RJ, Richards WO, O'Dorisio TM, Woltering EO, Williams S, Rice D, Abumrad NN: Efficacy of octreotide acetate in treatment of severe postgastrectomy dumping syndrome. Ann Surg 1990;212:678–687.
30 Mourad FH, Gorard D, Thillainayagam AV, Colin-Jones D, Farthing MJG: Effective treatment of diabetic diarrhoea with somatostatin analogue, octreotide. Gut 1992;33:1578–1580.
31 Nakabayashi H, Fujii S, Miwa U, Seta T, Takeda R: Marked improvement of diabetic diarrhea with the somatostatin analogue octreotide. Arch Intern Med 1994;154:1863–1867.
32 Walker JJ, Kaplan DS: Efficacy of the somatostatin analog octreotide in the treatment of two patients with refractory diabetic diarrhea. Am J Gastroenterol 1993;88:765–767.
33 Guarino A, Canani RB, Spagnuolo MI, Bisceglia M, Boccia MC, Rubino A: In vivo and in vitro efficacy of octreotide for treatment of enteric cryptosporidiosis. Dig Dis Sci 1988;43: 436–441.
34 Abbas Z, Moid I, Khan AH, Jafi SMW, Shah SHA, Abid S, Hamid S: Efficacy of octreotide in diarrhoea due to *Vibrio cholerae:* A randomized controlled trial. Ann Trop Med Parasitol 1996; 90:507–513.
35 Sharkey NMF, Kadden ML, Stabile BE: Severe posthemicolectomy diarrhea: Evaluation and treatment with SMS 201-995. Gastroenterology 1990;99:1144–1148.
36 Soudah HC, Hasler WL, Owyang CH: Effect of octreotide on intestinal motility and bacterial overgrowth in scleroderma. N Engl J Med 1991; 325:1461–1467.
37 Dean AP, Reed WD: Diarrhoea – An unrecognized hazard of coeliac plexus block. Aust NZ J Med 1991;21:47–48.
38 Smelt AHM, Meinders AE, Hoekman K, Noort WA, Keirse MJNC: Secretory diarrhea in villous adenoma of rectum: Effect of treatment with somatostatin and indomethacin. Prostaglandins 1992;43:657–572.

Digestion

Digestion 1999;60(suppl 2):47–52

Treatment of Acute Nonvariceal Upper Gastrointestinal Hemorrhage

R. Meier A.R. Wettstein

Gastroenterology Unit, University Hospital, Liestal, Switzerland

Key Words
Ulcer bleeding, incidence · Risk factors · Endoscopic treatment · Medical treatment · Somatostatin · Octreotide

Abstract
Hospitalization for nonvariceal upper gastrointestinal hemorrhage (UGIH) is still common with an incidence of 100/100,000 adults/year. Mortality rates range between 8 and 14%. The most common etiologies of acute UGIH are gastric and duodenal ulcers which are associated with older age, *Helicobacter pylori* gastritis and nonsteroidal anti-inflammatory drugs. Approximately 70% of UGIH stop spontaneously, 10% bleed continuously and about 20% rebleed in the first 24–72 h. Mortality and the probability of rebleeding have been related to the ulcers' stigmata (Forrest) and to a variety of clinical findings (hematemesis, low initial hemoglobin, signs of shock, coagulopathy and liver disease). It is well established that only patients with continued bleeding or with a risk of rebleeding benefit from endoscopic or medical treatment. Endoscopic treatment (including heater probe, bipolar electrocoagulation, laser and injection therapy) control active bleeding in up to 90% and reduce significantly the rates of further bleeding, the need for blood transfusions, hospital costs and emergency surgery. Medical treatment is still controversial although positive results for somatostatin and octreotide have been found. A meta-analysis including 1,829 patients from 14 randomized trials showed the relative risk for continued bleeding or rebleeding of 0.53 (95% CI, 0.43–0.63) in favor of somatostatin and octreotide. Interventional endoscopy is the first line of treatment for UGIH. Somatostatin and its analogue octreotide may be a useful adjunct to endoscopic management or alternative when endoscopy is unsuccessful, contraindicated or unavailable.

Hospitalization for acute nonvariceal upper gastrointestinal hemorrhage is still common. Recently published epidemiological data report an incidence of around 100/100,000 adults/year [1–3]. The incidence increases with age, with the highest proportion in those over 75 years [2]. The rate increases with age in both males and females. At all ages the incidence in males is higher than in females, except in the age group over 75 years [2]. Mortality rates range between 8 and 14% [2–4]. Mortality is higher in hospitalized and elderly patients due to a higher rate of comorbidity than in patients with an emergency hospital admission. Mortality in patients under 60 years without malignancy or organ failure is very low (<1%).

The most common etiologies of acute upper gastrointestinal hemorrhage are gastric and duodenal ulcers (table 1) [1]. Ulcers are associated with older age, *Helicobacter pylori* gastritis and nonsteroidal anti-inflammatory drug (NSAID) use [5, 6].

The natural history of ulcer bleeding is known from prospective and retrospective studies. Unfortunately these data are difficult to compare due to the use of nonstandardized terms. It is however known that approximately 70% of acute nonvariceal upper gastrointestinal hemorrhage stops spontaneously and 10% bleed continuously. Rebleeding in the first 24–72 h occurs in up to 20% [7, 8].

KARGER

Fax +41 61 306 12 34
E-Mail karger@karger.ch
www.karger.ch

0012–2823/99/0608–0047$17.50/0

Accessible online at:
http//BioMedNet.com/karger

Rémy Meier, MD
Gastroenterology Unit, University Hospital
Rheinstrasse 26
CH–4410 Liestal (Switzerland)
Tel. +41 61 925 21 87, Fax +41 61 925 28 04

Table 1. Etiology of upper gastrointestinal hemorrhage [1]

Etiology	n (%)
Peptic ulcer	
Duodenal ulcer	92 (35.7)
Gastric ulcer	62 (24.0)
Duodenal ulcer and gastric ulcer	3 (1.2)
Gastrojejunal ulcer	2 (0.8)
Mucosal erosive disease	
Gastritis	16 (6.2)
Duodenitis	4 (1.6)
Gastroduodenitis	7 (2.7)
Esophagitis	10 (3.9)
Esophageal varices	16 (6.2)
Miscellaneous	
Mallory-Weiss tear	9 (3.5)
Esophageal ulcer	4 (1.6)
Malignancy	4 (1.6)
Dieulafoy's lesion	3 (1.2)
Unknown	21 (8.1)
Total	258 (100)

Table 2. Bleeding activity according to Forrest [12]

Bleeding activity			Spontanous rebleeding rate
Forrest	I	Active bleeding	
	Ia	Active pulsation	90%
	Ib	Active oozing	30%
Forrest	II	Bleeding stigmata	
	IIa	Visible vessel	50%
	IIb	Clot	20%
	IIc	Black base	<5%
Forrest	III	No bleeding signs	
		Clear ulcer base	<5%

Table 3. Risk factors for rebleeding [18]

Risk factor	Yes	No
Stigmata (n = 79)	61%[1]	5%
Shock (n = 114)	66%[2]	2%
Stigmata and shock (n = 11)	79%	9%

1 Stigmata: Forrest IIa, 50%; Forrest IIb, 11%; Forrest IIc, 0%.
2 Pulse rate/systolic blood pressure: P > 100 beats/min/BP > 100 mm Hg: 18%; P > 100 beats/min/BP < 100 mm Hg: 48%.

There are well-known risk factors for continued or recurrent bleeding. The term 'rebleeding' should be restricted to those patients who either presented with hemodynamic stability at admission or in whom hemodynamic stability could be achieved within 24 h of admission and who rebleed after this time (24–72 h). Patients with signs of hemodynamic instability at admission and who could not be stabilized within 24 h should be classified as those with 'continued bleeding'. The target risk group for active treatment should be defined as those patients with continued bleeding or at high risk of rebleeding. Persistent or recurrent bleeding occurs in about 30% of the patients [9]. Improved diagnostic accuracy has not translated into a major reduction in the overall mortality rate from ulcer bleeding which has not changed much in the past decade. Mortality and the probability of rebleeding have been related to stigmata of hemorrhage and to a variety of clinical findings [10, 11]. Bleeding stigmata (table 2) according to the classification of Forrest were the first endoscopic predictive factors to assess the risk of rebleeding [12]. Active bleeding (pulsation or oozing) and visible vessels are associated with an increased risk of continued or recurrent bleeding. According to a recently published German multicenter trial, Ell et al. [13] found that active pulsatile bleeding occurred in 4%, oozing bleeding in 17% and a visible vessel was present in 16%. Among these endoscopic findings a visible vessel was a major indicator of uncontrolled or recurrent hemorrhage [14, 15]. The predictive value of a visible vessel in respect to rebleeding has been reported to a range from 50 to 100% [16, 17]. In addition, a visible vessel together with hemodynamic instability has a significantly increased probability of rebleeding (table 3) [10, 18].

Hematemesis and a low initial hemoglobin (< 11 g/dl) are both independent risk factors for persistent or recurrent bleeding, whereas liver disease and hematemesis are independent risk factors for intractable bleeding (table 4) [9]. The rate of mortality has been shown to correspond with these risk factors. Terdiman et al. [9] found mortality rates of 14.3% in patients with and of 1% in patients without further bleeding. In patients who did not present with hematemesis, liver disease, coagulopathy, hypotension and low initial hemoglobin, the frequency of further bleeding and mortality was 0%. Furthermore, the risk of rebleeding significantly increases with age, especially in patients with hemodynamic instability [19].

From these data it is possible to select patients with a high risk (of continued or recurrent bleeding) for active treatment on the basis of clinical and endoscopic findings. Clinical trials should only be performed on these strictly

Table 4. Risk factors for persistent or recurrent and intractable bleeding [9]

Risk factor	OR (95% CI)	p value
Persistent or recurrent bleeding		
Hematemesis	5.7 (2.4–13.1)	0.001
Low hemoglobin	0.8 (0.7–0.96)	0.01
Interactable bleeding		
Liver disease	6.0 (2.0–18.4)	0.002
Hematemesis	3.7 (1.2–11.0)	0.008

selected patients in whom the chance of spontaneous cessation of bleedings are as low as possible. It is proven that only these subgroups of patients will benefit from active treatment. The numerous previous published trials which fail to show a beneficial effect of endoscopic intervention may reflect inappropriate patient selection.

Treatment of Acute Nonvariceal Upper Gastrointestinal Bleeding

Endoscopic Treatment

It is now well established that endoscopic interventions are successful in stopping active hemorrhage. Untreated active hemorrhage is associated with continued bleeding or rebleeding rates of 80–100% [20]. Endoscopic treatment reduces significantly the rates of further bleeding, the need for blood transfusions, hospital costs and emergency surgery [21]. Endoscopic therapy including heater probe, bipolar electrocoagulation, laser and injection therapy can control active bleeding in up to 90% of patients. In 1989, the NIH consensus panel on therapeutic endoscopy and gastrointestinal bleeding recommended that patients with clinical features associated with a high risk of recurrent bleeding or endoscopic evidence of active bleeding or visible blood vessels should undergo endoscopic therapy [22]. Interventional endoscopy is now considered the gold standard in the acute management of bleeding ulcer disease. Review of the literature suggests that heater probe, bipolar electrocoagulation, laser and injection therapy are comparable in their safety and efficacy [23–30]. Many endoscopists prefer injection therapy with epinephrine, with or without concomitant ethoxysclerol because of its convenience.

Medical Treatment

Although endoscopy treatment is very effective, there are still a number of patients in which bleeding cannot be controlled. For this reason a variety of drugs including H_2-antagonists, proton-pump inhibitors, tranexamic acid, somatostatin and its analogues have been used to control the bleeding further. Neither oral nor intravenous H_2-antagonists have been shown to significantly alter clinical outcomes [31, 32]. Similarly, tranexamic acid has also been shown to be ineffective [33, 34]. In a recently performed study by Lin et al. [35], significantly fewer rebleeding episodes were seen with omeprazole as compared to H_2-antagonists on days 3 and 14 although the length of hospital stay, the number of patients requiring surgery and mortality rates were not significantly influenced.

Somatostatin, an endogenous peptide that reduces splanchnic blood flow and gastrointestinal motility, inhibits basal and stimulated gastric acid, pepsin and gastrin secretion and may have gastric cytoprotective effects, was proposed for the treatment of upper gastrointestinal bleeding [36–48]. The efficacy of somatostatin in the control of nonvariceal upper gastrointestinal hemorrhage is uncertain. Eight trials [49–56] showed positive effects whilst 4 trials [57–60] showed no favorable effect as compared to H_2-antagonists or placebo. The inconsistency between these trials may be explained by small sample size and clinical heterogeneity of the study groups.

Octreotide, an 8-amino-acid synthetic analogue of somatostatin was found to be more selective with a greater pharmacological activity and a longer half-life than the native molecule. Furthermore, the bioavailability after administration of octreotide is similar for intravenous infusion or subcutaneous injections [61, 62]. The rationale for using octreotide in the treatment of upper gastrointestinal bleeding is the combination of pronounced inhibition of gastric acid secretion and decrease of splanchnic blood flow [63]. An open pilot trial in patients with acute bleeding due to gastric or duodenal ulcer showed that octreotide was well tolerated and may be useful in arresting bleeding and preventing rebleeding [64]. The first double-blind, placebo-controlled multicenter trial however showed that octreotide was no more effective in arresting ulcer bleeding and preventing rebleeding than placebo (70.6 vs. 69.6%) [65]. Surgery rates, blood transfusion requirements and the time before bleeding stopped were also not different between the two groups. A retrospective subgroup analysis according to age, sex, localization of the ulcer, severity of bleeding and arterial spurting vs. oozing showed homogeneity and did not allow identification of a subgroup that might benefit from treatment with octreotide. This study has been criticized for the high response in the placebo group (70.6%) which suggests that patients with a high risk of continued or recurrent

Table 5. Octreotide in acute peptic ulcer bleeding (PR, controlled trial) [66]

	n	Bleeding stop	Endoscopic therapy or surgery	Blood transfusion	Deaths, n
Octreotide and ranitidine	42	35 (83%)	7	250 ml (0–5,000)	2
Ranitidine	42	23 (55%)	17	1,000 ml (0–8,000)	4
p value		$p<0.01$	$p<0.05$	$p<0.05$	NS

Table 6. Somatostatin or octreotide compared with H_2-antagonists or placebo in upper gastrointestinal hemorrhage – a meta-Analysis [67] (14 randomized clinical trials ($n=1,829$): 12 somatostatin and 2 octreotide)

Outcome measure	Trials, n	Relative risk (95% CI)
Continued or rebleeding		
All	14	0.53 (0.43–0.63)
Investigator blind	7	0.73 (0.64–0.81)
Peptic ulcer	8	0.48 (0.39–0.59)
Nonpeptic ulcer	4	0.62 (0.99–1.02)
Surgery		
Investigator blind	7	0.94 (0.87–1.0)

bleeding were not selected. Furthermore, a mean hemoglobin value of >11 g/dl indicated that the bleeding was not severe. On the other hand, a recently published study by Lin et al. [66], comparing intravenous octreotide and ranitidine in patients with active peptic ulcer bleeding or nonbleeding vessels, found a hemostatis rate in 84 and 55%, respectively ($p<0.01$) (table 5). Volume of blood transfused, number of patients receiving aggressive management (endoscopic hemostatis or operation) and hospital stay were significantly fewer in the octreotide group. No significant side effects were found in the octreotide group.

In 1997, Imperiale and Birgisson [67] performed a meta-analysis including 1,829 patients from 14 randomized trials. They included 12 trials with somatostatin and 2 with octreotide and extracted data on outcome including continued bleeding, rebleeding during the treatment period, need for surgery and the transfusion requirements. The relative risk for continued bleeding or rebleeding was 0.53 (95% Cl, 0.43–0.63) in favor of somatostatin and octreotide. Active treatment was efficacious for peptic ulcer bleeding with a trend toward efficacy for nonpeptic ulcer bleeding. Although the overall results suggested a decreased need for surgery in the somatostatin group, a subgroup analysis of investigator-blinded trials revealed a more modest effect that was not statistically significant (table 6). In 7 trials the number of packed red blood cell transfusions required were reported. Among these trials no statistically significant difference between the somatostatin and the control group were found, although the weighted difference in transfusion requirement was 1.1 unit less for somatostatin. Five additional trials provided median or mean transfusion requirements without a variance measure [50, 56, 58, 65, 66]. In 4 [50, 56, 58, 66] of the 5 trials the transfusion requirement was lower for patients receiving somatostatin or octreotide than for controls. In 3 of these 4 trials the difference was statistically significant [50, 56, 66]. Although these overall results suggest that somatostatin or octreotide significantly reduces the risk of continued bleeding and the need for surgery, these results were derived from heterogeneous studies.

Future Strategies for Nonvariceal Upper Gastrointestinal Hemorrhage

Interventional endoscopy is the gold standard in the acute management of upper gastrointestinal bleeding due to peptic ulcer disease although it is still unsuccessful in 5–10% of cases. Somatostatin and its analogue octreotide reduce the risk of continued or recurrent bleeding due to peptic ulcer disease and may be a useful adjunct to endoscopic management or alternative when endoscopy is unsuccessful, contraindicated or unavailable. Unfortunately no trials have been published using somatostatin or octreotide before endoscopy or as a combination with endoscopic treatment. Further studies should clarify whether such strategies are more successful.

References

1 Longstreth GF: Epidemiology of hospitalization for acute upper gastrointestinal hemorrhage: A population-based study. Am J Gastroenterol 1995;90:206–210.

2 Rockall TA, Logan RFA, Devlin HB, Northfield TC: Incidence of and mortality from acute gastrointestinal haemorrhage in the United Kingdom. BMJ 1995;311:222–226.

3 Yavorski RT, Wong RK, Maydonovitch C, Battin LS, Furnia A, Amundson DE: Analysis of 3,294 cases of upper gastrointestinal bleeding in military medical facilities. Am J Gastroenterol 1995;90:568–573.

4 Rockall TA, Logan RFA, Devlin HB, Northfield TC: Variation in outcome after acute upper gastrointestinal hemorrhage. Lancet 1995;346:346–350.

5 Armstrong CP, Blower AL: Non-steroidal anti-inflammatory drugs and life-threatening complications of peptic ulceration. Gut 1987;28:527–532.

6 Henriksson AE, Edman AC, Nilsson I, Bergqvist D, Waldström T: *Helicobacter pylori* and the relation to other risk factors in patients with acute bleeding peptic ulcer. Scand J Gastroenterol 1998;33:1030–1033.

7 Gyr K, Kayasseh L: Indikation und Verfahrenswahl; in Siewert JR, Blum AI, Farthmann EC, Lankisch PG (eds): Interdisziplinäre Gastroenterologie. Notfalltherapie. Berlin, Springer, 1982, pp 233–245.

8 Collins R, Langman M: Treatment with histamine H_2-antagonists in acute upper gastrointestinal hemorrhage. Implications of randomized trials. N Engl J Med 1985;313:660–666.

9 Terdiman JP, Ostroff JW: Risk of persistent or recurrent and intractable upper gastrointestinal bleeding in the era of therapeutic endoscopy. Am J Gastroenterol 1997;92:1805–1811.

10 Katschinski B, Logan R, Davies J, Faulkner G, Pearson J, Langman M: Prognostic factors in upper gastrointestinal bleeding. Dig Dis Sci 1994;39:706–712.

11 Rockall TA, Logan RFA, Devlin HB, Northfield TC: Selection of patients for early discharge or outpatient care after acute upper gastrointestinal hemorrhage. Lancet 1996;347:1138–1140.

12 Forrest JAH, Finlayson NDC, Shearman DJC: Endoscopy in gastrointestinal bleeding. Lancet 1974;ii:394–397.

13 Ell C, Hagenmüller F, Schmitt W, Riemann JF, Hahn EG, Hohenberger W: Multizentrische prospektive Untersuchung zum aktuellen Stand der Therapie der Ulcusblutung in Deutschland. Dtsch Med Wschr 1995;120:3–9.

14 Griffiths WJ, Neumann DA, Welsh JD: The visible vessel as an indicator of uncontrolled or recurrent gastrointestinal hemorrhage. N Engl J Med 1979;300:1411–1413.

15 Storey DW, Bown SG, Swain CP, Salmon PR, Kirkham JS, Northfield TC: Endoscopic prediction of recurrent bleeding in peptic ulcers. N Engl J Med 1981;305:915–916.

16 Vallon AG, Cotton PB, Laurence BH, Miro JRA, Oses JCS: Randomised trial of endoscopic argon laser photocoagulation in bleeding peptic ulcers. Gut 1981;22:228–233.

17 MacLeod A, Mills PR: Factors identifying the probability of further haemorrhage after acute upper gastrointestinal haemorrhage. Br J Surg 1982;69:256–258.

18 Bornman C, Theodorou NA, Shuttleworth RD, Essel HP, Marks IN: Importance of hypovolaemic shock and endoscopic signs in predicting recurrent haemorrhage from peptic ulceration: A prospective evaluation. Br Med J 1985;291:245–247.

19 Hasselgren G, Carlsson J, Lind T, Schaffalitzky de Muckadell O, Lundell L: Risk factors for rebleeding and fatal outcome in elderly patients with acute peptic ulcer bleeding. Eur J Gastroenterol Hepatol 1998;10:667–672.

20 Pimpl W, Boeckl O, Waclawiczek HW: Estimation of the mortality rate of patients with severe gastroduodenal hemorrhage with the aid of a new scoring system. Endoscopy 1987;19:101–106.

21 Cook DJ, Guyatt GH, Salena BJ, Laine LA: Endoscopic therapy for acute nonvariceal upper gastrointestinal hemorrhage: A meta-anlaysis. Gastroenterology 1992;102:139–148.

22 NIH: Consensus Conference: Therapeutic endoscopy and bleeding ulcers. JAMA 1989;262:1369–1372.

23 Chung SCS, Leung JWC, Steele RJC, Crofts TJ, Li AKC: Endoscopic injection of adrenaline for acitvely bleeding ulcers: A randomised trial. BMJ 1988;296:1631–1633.

24 Lin HJ, Lee FY, Kang WM, Tsai YT, Lee SD, Lee CH: Heat probe thermocoagulation and pure alcohol injection in massive peptic ulcer haemorrhage: A prospective, randomised controlled trial. Gut 1990;31:753–757.

25 Chung SCS, Leung JWC, Sung KKL, Lo KK, Li AKC: Injection or heat probe for bleeding ulcer. Gastroenterology 1991;100:33–37.

26 Chung SC, Leung JWC, Leong HT, Lo KK, Li AKC: Adding a sclerosant to endoscopic epinephrine injection in actively bleeding ulcers: A randomized trial. Gastrointest Endosc 1993;39:611–615.

27 Lin HJ, Perng CL, Lee SD: Is sclerosant injection mandatory after an epinephrine injection for arrest of peptic ulcer haemorrhage? A prospective, randomised, comparative study. Gut 1993;34:1182–1185.

28 Lin HJ, Perng CL, Lee FY: Endoscopic injection for the arrest of peptic ulcer hemorrhage: Final results of a prospective, randomized comparative trial. Gastrointest Endosc 1993;39:15–19.

29 Saeed ZA, Winchester CB, Michaletz PA, Woods KL, Graham DY: A scoring system to predict rebleeding after endoscopic therapy of nonvariceal upper gastrointestinal hemorrhage, with a comparison of heat probe and ethanol injection. Am J Gastroenterol 1993;88:1842–1849.

30 Llach J, Bordas JM, Salmeron JM, Panes J, Garcia-Pagan JC, Feu F, Navasa Mondelo F, Pique JM, Mas A, Ters J, Rodes J: A prospective randomized trial of heater probe thermocoagulation versus injection therapy in peptic ulcer hemorrhage. Gastrointest Endosc 1996;43:117–120.

31 Liebermann D: Gastrointestinal bleeding: Initial management. Gastroenterol Clin North Am 1993;22:723–736.

32 Laine L: Rolling review: Upper gastrointestinal bleeding. Aliment Pharmacol Ther 1993;7:207–232.

33 Cormack F, Jouhar AJ, Chakrabarti RR, Fearnley GR: Tranexamic acid in upper gastrointestinal haemorrhage. Lancet 1973;i:1207–1208.

34 Barer D, Ogilvie A, Henry D, Dornfield M, Coggon D, French S, Ellis S, Atkins M, Langman M: Cimetidine and tranexamic acid in treatment of acute upper gastrointestinal-tract bleeding. N Engl J Med 1983;26:1571–1575.

35 Lin HJ, Lo WC, Lee FY, Lee SD: A prospective randomized comparative trial showing that omeprazole prevents rebleeding in bleeding peptic ulcer patients after successful endoscopic therapy. DDW Abstract 1771, 1997.

36 Bosch J, Kravetz D, Rodes J: Effect of somatostatin on hepatic and systemic hemodynamics in patients with cirrhosis of the liver. Comparison with vasopressin. Gastroenterology 1981;80:518–525.

37 Bloom SR, Mortimer CH, Thorner MO, Besser GM, Hall R, Gomez-Pan A: Inhibition of gastrin and gastric-acid secretion by growth-hormone release-inhibiting hormone. Lancet 1974;ii:1106–1109.

38 Johansson C, Aly A: Stimulation of gastric mucus output by somatostatin in man. Eur J Clin Invest 1982;12:37–39.

39 Bloom SR, Russel RCG, Barros-D'sa AAJ, Baron JH, Besser GM, Hall R, Coy H, Kastin AJ, Scholly AV: Inhibition of gastrin and gastric acid by growth hormone inhibiting hormone. Gut 1975;16:396–400.

40 Arnold R, Creutzfeldt W: Hemmung der Pentagastrin-induzierten Säuresekretion des Magens beim Menschen durch Somatostatin. Dtsch Med Wochenschr 1975;100:1014–1016.

41 Johansson C, Wissen O, Kollberg B, Uvnäs-Wallensten K, Efendic S: Effects of intragastrically administered somatostatin on basal and pentagastrin stimulated gastric acid secretion in man. Acta Physiol Scand 1978;104:232–234.

42 Whitehouse I, Beglinger Ch, Fried M, Gyr K: The effect of octapeptide somatostatin analogue (SMS 201-995) and Somatostatin-14 (SST-14) on pentagastrin-stimulated gastric acid secretion: A comparative study in man. Hepatogastroenterologica 1984;31:227–229.

43 Loud FB, Holst JJ, Egense E, Petersen B, Christiansen J: Is somatostatin a humoral regulator of the endocrine pancreas and gastric acid secretion in man? Gut 1985;26:445–449.

44 Schrumpf E, Vatn MH, Hanssen KF, Myren J: A small dose of somatostatin inhibits the pentagastrin-stimulated gastric secretion of acid, pepsin and intrinsic factor in man. Clin Endocrinol 1978;8:391–395.
45 Thomas WEG: Somatostatin – The long lost antral chalone. Med Hypoth 1980;6:919–927.
46 Wahren J, Felig P: Influence of somatostatin on carbohydrate disposal and absorption in diabetes mellitus. Lancet 1976;ii:1213–1216.
47 Arnold R, Lankisch PG: Somatostatin and the gastrointestinal tract. Clin Gastroenterol 1980; 9:733–753.
48 Sonnenberg GE, Keller U, Perruchoud A, Burckhardt D, Gyr K: Effect of somatostatin on splanchnic hemodynamics in patients with cirrhosis of the liver and in normal subjects. Gastroenterology 1981;80:526–532.
49 Kayasseh L, Gyr K, Keller U, Stalder GA, Wall M: Somatostatin and cimetidine in peptic-ulcer haemorrhage: A randomised controlled trial. Lancet 1980;i:844–846.
50 Basile M, Celi S, Parisi A, Castiglione N, Parisi S: Somatostatin in the treatment of severe gastrointestinal bleeding from peptic origin. A multicentric controlled trial. Ital J Surg Sci 1984; 14:31–35.
51 Coraggio F, Scarpato P, Spina M, Lombardi S: Somatostatin and ranitidine in the control of iatrogenic haemorrhage of the upper gastrointestinal tract. Br Med J 1984;289:224.
52 Magnusson I, Ihre T, Johansson C, Seligson U, Törngren S, Uvnäs-Moberg K: Randomised double-blind trial of somatostatin in the treatment of massive upper gastrointestinal hemorrhage. Gut 1985;26:221–226.
53 Antonioli A, Gandolfo M, Rigo GP, Bianchi Porro G, Cheli R, Brancato F, Lazzaroni M, Parodi MC, Maringhini A, Raimundo S, Manenti F: Somatostatin and cimetidine in the control of acute upper gastrointestinal bleeding. A controlled multicenter study. Hepatogastroenterology 1986;33:71–74.
54 Torres AJ, Landa I, Hernandez F, Jover JM, Suarez A, Arias J, Cuberas R, Santoyo J, Fernandez R, Colleja J, Nisa E, Rodriquez JL, Moreno E, Balibrea JL: Somatostatin in the treatment of severe upper gastrointestinal bleeding. A multicentre controlled trial. Br J Surg 1986;73:786–789.
55 Coraggio F, Bertini G, Catalano A, Scarpato P, Gualdieri L: Clinical controlled trial of somatostatin with ranitidine and placebo in the control of peptic hemorrhage of the upper gastrointestinal tract. Digestion 1989;43:190–195.
56 Tulassay Z, Gupta R, Papp J, Bodnar A: Somatostatin versus cimetidine in the treatment of actively bleeding duodenal ulcer: A prospective, randomized controlled trial. Am J Gastroenterol 1989;84:6–9.
57 Galmiche JP, Cassigneul J, Faivre J, Tranvouez JL, Ouvry D, Colin R, Pascal JP, Klepping C: Somatostatin in peptic ulcer bleeding – Results of a double-blind controlled trial. Int J Clin Pharmacol Res 1983;3:379–387.
58 Somerville KW, Henry DA, Davies JG, Hine KR, Hawkey CJ, Langman MJ: Somatostatin in the treatment of haemorrhage and melaena. Lancet 1985;i:130–132.
59 Basso N, Bagarani M, Bracci F, Cucchiara G, Gizzonio D, Grassini G, Percoco M, Procacciante F, Toti F: Ranitidine and somatostatin. Their effects on bleeding from the upper gastrointestinal tract. Arch Surg 1986;121:833–835.
60 Saperas E, Piqué JM, Pérez-Ayuso R, Fuster F, Terés J, Bordas JM, Rodes J: Somatostatin compared with cimetidine in the treatment of bleeding peptic ulcer without visible vessel. Aliment Pharmacol Ther 1988;2:153–159.
61 Bauer W, Briner U, Doepfner W, Haller R, Hugnenin R, Marbach P, Petcher TJ, Pless J: Octreotide: A very potent and selective octapeptide analogue of somatostatin with prolonged action. Life Sci 1982;31:1133–1140.
62 Kutz K, Nüesch E, Rosenthaler J: Pharmacokinetics of SMS 201-995 in healthy subjects. Scand J Gastroenterol 1986;21(suppl):65–72.
63 Wahren J, Eriksson LS: The influence of a long-acting somatostatin analogue on splanchnic haemodynamics and metabolism in healthy subjects and patients with liver cirrhosis. Scand J Gastroenterol 1986;21(suppl 119):103–108.
64 Christiansen J, Yotis A: The role of somatostatin and a long-acting analogue, SMS 201-995, in acute bleeding due to peptic ulceration. Scand J Gastroenteol 1986;21(suppl 119):109–114.
65 Christiansen J, Ottenjann R, Von Arx F: Placebo-controlled trial with the somatostatin analogue SMS 201–995 in peptic ulcer bleeding. Gastroenterology 1989;97:568–574.
66 Lin HJ, Perng CL, Wang K, Lee CH, Lee SD: Octreotide for arrest of peptic ulcer hemorrhage – A prospective, randomized controlled trial. Hepatogastroenterology 1995;42:856–860.
67 Imperiale TF, Birgisson S: Somatostatin or octreotide compared with H_2-antagonists and placebo in the management of acute nonvariceal upper gastrointestinal hemorrhage: A metaanalysis. Ann Intern Med 1997;127:12:1062–1071.

Digestion

Digestion 1999;60(suppl 2):53–56

Role of Octreotide and Somatostatin in the Treatment of Intestinal Fistulae

G. Dorta

Division of Gastroenterology CHUV/PMU, University Hospital, Lausanne, Switzerland

Key Words

Intestinal fistulae · Octreotide · Somatostatin · Fistula closure rate

Abstract

Intestinal fistulae usually arise as a complication of abdominal surgery. Its treatment is complex and intestinal fistula-related morbidity and mortality is high. Fistula closure rates under conservative medical treatment vary between 24 and 72%. Octreotide and somatostatin reduce gastrointestinal, biliary and pancreatic secretion and increase intestinal water and electrolyte absorption. In recent years, octreotide and somatostatin have been associated with conservative medical treatment for patients with intestinal fistulae. Four placebo-controlled studies have been published within the past 6 years. The interpretation of their results is difficult because patient collectives were small and heterogeneous. In one study, somatostatin decreased fistula-related complications when compared to placebo, and in another study, octreotide decreased the healing time of intestinal fistulae and the time patients required total parenteral nutrition when compared to placebo. In contrast, the fistula closure rate, hospitalization time and mortality were not influenced by the use of octreotide or somatostatin in conservative medical treatment. In conclusion, octreotide and somatostatin actually cannot be recommended in the treatment of intestinal fistulae in settings outside of controlled trials.

Introduction

Intestinal fistulae are rare but serious deseases. They usually arise as a complication of abdominal surgery, abdominal trauma, Crohn's disease, intra-abdominal abscesses, radiation therapy, chemotherapy and neoplasia. Most intestinal fistulae are due to abdominal surgery. Some 75–85% of small bowel fistulae are complications of abdominal surgery [1–3]. The complications strongly correlate with the anatomical site of the fistula, the volume and the composition of the fistula output, as well as the underlying pathology. Conservative treatment consists of correcting water and electrolyte imbalances and repleting ongoing losses, protecting the skin around the fistula, treatment and prevention of infection, and the restoration and maintenance of the nutritional status with intravenous hyperalimentation.

Under conservative medical treatment, the spontaneous closure rate of intestinal fistulae varies between 24 and 72% within 27–39 days, and the mortality lies between 5 and 29%, predominantly secondary to infections [1, 4–6]. Despite progress in medical management, the mortality rate has not changed during the past 30 years [6] and the time to closure under conservative medical treatment is long and often associated with all the inconveniences and complications of prolonged hospitalization. Therefore, new treatment modalities for intestinal fistulae are warranted. New hope was offered by treating intestinal fistulae with the agents octreotide and somatostatin. These two substances reduce gastrointestinal, biliary and pancreatic secretions, decrease gut motility, and increase water and electrolyte absorption in the small intestine [7–10]. The fistula output can thus be reduced

KARGER

Fax +41 61 306 12 34
E-Mail karger@karger.ch
www.karger.ch

0012–2823/99/0608–0053$17.50/0

Accessible online at:
http//BioMedNet.com/karger

G. Dorta
Division of Gastroenetrology CHUV/PMU
BH 10 CHUV, CH–1011 Lausanne (Switzerland)
Tel. + +41 021 314 06 80, Fax + +41 021 314 07 07
E-Mail gian.dorta@chuv.hospvd.ch

Table 1. Effectiveness of octreotide/somatostatin in placebo-controlled trials

Group (first author)	Year	Patients with intestinal/ other fistulae, n	Active drug	Effectiveness on:			
				closure rate	healing time	complication rate	mortality
Torres [20]	1992	33/7	Somatostatin	NS	NS	Pos	NS
Hernandez-Aranda [21]	1996	56/43	Octreotide	NS	Pos	–	NS
Scott [22]	1993	19	Octreotide	NS	NS	NS	NS
Sancho [23]	1995	26/5	Octreotide	NS	NS	NS	NS

– = Not evaluated; NS = no statistical difference between placebo and active drug; Pos = positive effect of active drug.

by both agents, and one could speculate that the two agents might have a beneficial effect on fistula closure. The effects on gastrointestinal secretion and absorption evoked by octreotide and somatostatin do not clinically differ, but octreotide has a 30- to 100-fold longer elimination half-life time than somatostatin [11]. This fact simplifies the treatment modalities.

Intestinal fistulae of Crohn's disease had occasionally been treated with octreotide. Within the perspective of the excellent results afforded by antitumor necrosis factor-α treatment, octreotide treatment may no longer have a place in the treatment of fistulae associated with Crohn's disease [12, 13].

Literature Review: Octreotide and Somatostatin in the Treatment of Intestinal Fistulae

The first clinical trial of octreotide in fistulae of the small intestine was published in 1987 [10]. In a blind crossover trial which lasted 4 days, the authors demonstrated that the fistula output could be dramatically reduced by the administration of octreotide. Within the past 11 years, a large number of papers covering the treatment of intestinal fistulae with octreotide or somatostatin have been published. Unfortunately, there were only a few prospective, controlled studies. Furthermore, there was no publication that compared the efficacy of somatostatin versus octreotide in the treatment of intestinal fistulae in a randomized study.

The multiple case reports concerning octreotide in the treatment of intestinal fistulae are not reviewed because they provide only stage IV evidence regarding the efficacy of octreotide treatment in intestinal fistulae.

Furthermore, several patient series and multiple case reports concerning octreotide in the treatment of intestinal fistulae have been published in the last years. The most important series shows fistula closure rates ranging from 43 to 75% within 6–37 days. These results are not different from the healing rates observed under conservative medical treatment. The patient number varies between 14 and 40 patients. In all these studies, octreotide had been administered in a dosage of 300 μg daily, until fistula closure [14–17].

Complications of octreotide treatment reported in these series were not frequent and mostly of a minor nature: pain at the injection sites occurred in 15–30% of the patients [14, 17]. One patient, who had previously received somatostatin treatment, developed a mild hypersensitivity reaction that could be controlled with oral antihistamines [17].

In a retrospective study, the treatment with octreotide significantly increased the fistula closure rate and decreased the mortality rate when compared to the control subjects. Unfortunately, in this study, as well, the data analysis did not separately treat patients with intestinal and pancreatic fistulae [18]. Another retrospective study compared four different treatment modalities: wound care only, conservative treatment including total parenteral nutrition, conservative treatment including total parenteral nutrition in association with an octreotide dosage ranging from 150 μg to 1,500 μg, and surgical treatment. The number of patients in each treatment group was very small and did not permit any statistical analysis. However, patients treated with octreotide or surgery had a better fistula closure rate when compared to the other two treatment modalities [19].

Within the past 6 years, there have been four placebo-controlled trials published that followed a conservative medical treatment using either octreotide or somatostatin (table 1). In a randomized, placebo-controlled trial using somatostatin (250 μg/h during 20 days), Torres et al. [20] treated 33 patients with intestinal fistulae and 7 patients with pancreatic fistulae. The interpretation of this study is difficult because the cases of intestinal fistulae and pancreatic fistulae were not analyzed separately. Closure rate, healing time and mortality were similar in the placebo and in the somatostatin group. However, more complications occurred in the group treated with placebo than in the somatostatin group (68 vs. 35%, $p < 0.05$). Two patients undergoing somatostatin treatment developed hyperglycemia, which was controlled with insulin.

In the study by Hernandez-Aranda et al. [21], octreotide was given in a dosage of 100 µg t.i.d. in patients with enterocutanous fistulae. Fifty-six of the 99 patients had small bowel fistulae, but unfortunately, these cases had not been evaluated separately. Overall, fistula closure rate, hospital stay and mortality rates were similar in the placebo and octreotide groups. Healing time in case of spontaneous closure of the fistula (18 vs. 27 days, $p = 0.002$) and the time patients required total parenteral nutrition (22 vs. 29 days, $p = 0.04$) were shorter in the octreotide group than in the placebo group.

Two other placebo-controlled trials including 19 and 26 patients with intestinal fistulas, respectively, showed no significant differences with respect to closure rate, healing time, complications and mortality [22, 23]. In these studies, octreotide 100 µg t.i.d. was administered during 12 and 20 days, respectively. In the trial by Sancho et al. [23], 4 of the 14 patients in the octreotide group had local pain at the injection sites, but no major adverse effects were reported.

Discussion and Conclusions

The evaluation of the efficacy of octreotide or somatostatin in the treatment of intestinal fistulae is difficult. There are many published patient series and case reports but only a few published controlled studies comparing octreotide or somatostatin versus placebo in the treatment of intestinal fistulae. Furthermore, these controlled studies have had very heterogeneous and small patient collectives, and often included patients with pancreatic fistulae. Unfortunately, analysis of the outcomes has not been carried out separately for the patients with intestinal fistulae. In all these studies, the fistula closure rate, mortality rate and hospitalization time were not decreased by octreotide or somatostatin treatment when compared to placebo. However, two controlled studies reported beneficial effects of octreotide and somatostatin. The study by Torres et al. [20] showed a lower complication rate in the group treated with somatostatin when compared with placebo, and the study by Hernandez-Aranda et al. [21] showed a faster healing time and patients in the octreotide group needed total parenteral nutrition for a shorter time than did those with placebo. Further prospective, controlled studies of octreotide treatment in patients with intestinal fistulae are needed to confirm the positive results obtained in the two cited studies. Ideally, these studies would include only patients having intestinal fistulae as well as a larger number of patients than those included in the published studies.

The multiple case reports, patients series and the two retrospective studies [18, 19] give only 'stage III and IV' evidence of the effectiveness of octreotide and somatostatin. In all the reviewed publications, side effects of octreotide and somatostatin were not frequent and always of a minor nature.

In conclusion, based on the published controlled trials and its endpoints, octreotide and somatostatin actually cannot be recommended for the treatment of intestinal fistulae and further prospective studies might confirm the positive preliminary results obtained in two controlled studies. However, there is 'stage III and IV' evidence regarding the effectiveness of octreotide and somatostatin. Patients with intestinal fistulae can be treated with octreotide or somatostatin, but treatment should be stopped if the fistula output does not decrease in the first 48 h of the treatment. The treatment of patients with high output fistulae may be simplified by octreotide or somatostatin treatment reducing depletion of fluid, electrolytes and protein.

References

1 Aguirre A, Fischer JE, Welch CE: The role of surgery and hyperalimentation in therapy of gastrointestinal-cutaneous fistulae. Ann Surg 1974;180:393–401.

2 Rinsema W, Gouma DJ, von Meyenfeldt MF, van der Linden CJ, Soeters PB: Primary conservative management of external small-bowel fistulas. Changing composition of fistula series? Acta Chir Scand 1990;156:457–462.

3 Kuvshinoff BW, Brodish RJ, McFadden DW, Fischer JE: Serum transferrin as a prognostic indicator of spontaneous closure and mortality in gastrointestinal cutaneous fistulae. Ann Surg 1993;217:615–622.

4 Sitges-Serra A, Jaurrieta E, Sitges-Creus A: Management of postoperative enterocutaneous fistulas: The roles of parenteral nutrition and surgery. Br J Surg 1982;69:147–150.

5 Soeters PB, Ebeid AM, Fischer JE: Review of 404 patients with gastrointestinal fistulas. Impact of parenteral nutrition. Ann Surg 1979;190:189–202.

6 Berry SM, Fischer JE: Enterocutaneous fistulas. Curr Probl Surg 1994;31:469–566.

7 Fuessl HS, Carolan G, Williams G, Bloom SR: Effect of a long-acting somatostatin analogue (SMS 201–995) on postprandial gastric emptying of ^{99m}Tc-tin colloid and mouth-to-caecum transit time in man. Digestion 1987;36:101–107.

8 Moller N, Petrany G, Cassidy D, Sheldon WL, Johnston DG, Laker MF: Effects of the somatostatin analogue SMS 201–995 (Sandostatin) on mouth-to-caecum transit time and absorption of fat and carbohydrates in normal man. Clin Sci 1988;75:345–350.

9 Lembcke B, Creutzfeldt W, Schleser S, Ebert R, Shaw C, Koop I: Effect of the somatostatin analogue Sandostatin (SMS 201–995) on gastrointestinal, pancreatic and biliary function and hormone release in normal men. Digestion 1987;36:108–124.

10 Nubiola-Calonge P, Badia JM, Sancho J, Gil MJ, Segura M, Sitges-Serra A: Blind evaluation of the effect of octreotide (SMS 201–995), a somatostatin analogue, on small-bowel fistula output. Lancet 1987;ii:672–674.

11 Gyr KE, Meier R: Pharmacodynamic effects of Sandostatin in the gastrointestinal tract. Digestion 1993;54(suppl 1):14–19.

12 Bouma G, Poen AC, Garcia-Gonzalez MA, Schreuder GMT, Felt-Bersma RJF, Meuwissen SGM, Pena AS: HLA-DRB1*03, but not the TNFA-308 promoter gene polymorphism, confers protection against fistulising Crohn's disease. Immunogenetics 1998;47:451–455.

13 Van Hogezand RA, Verspaget HW: The future role of anti-tumour necrosis factor-alpha products in the treatment of Crohn's disease. Drugs 1998;56:299–305.

14 Paran H, Neufeld D, Kaplan O, Klausner J, Freund U: Octreotide for treatment of postoperative alimentary tract fistulas. World J Surg 1995;19:430–433.

15 Spiliotis J, Briand D, Gouttebel MC, Astre C, Louer B, Saint-Aubert B, Kalfarentzos F, Androulakis J, Joyeux H: Treatment of fistulae of the gastrointestinal tract with total parenteral nutrition and octreotide in patients with carcinoma. Surg Gynecol Obstet 1993;176:575–580.

16 Scott NA, Finnegan S, Irving MH: Octreotide and gastrointestinal fistulae. Digestion 1990; 45(suppl 1):66–70.

17 Nubiola-Calonge P, Badia JM, Martinez-Rodenas F, Gil MJ, Segura M, Sancho J, Sitges-Serra A: Treatment of 27 postoperative enterocutaneous fistulas with the long half-life somatostatin analogue SMS 201–995. Ann Surg 1989;210:56–58.

18 Munteanu D, Duca S, Vlad L, Paraian I, Toganel D, Iancu C, Pop F, Radu H, Puia C, Bala O, Bud O, Nagy Z, Leuca D, Bordei R, Popazu R: Sandostatin treatment in postoperative external digestive fistulae. Chirurgia (Bucur) 1998; 93:13–21.

19 Borison DI, Bloom AD, Pritchard TJ: Treatment of enterocutaneous and colocutaneous fistulas with early surgery or somatostatin analog. Dis Colon Rectum 1992;35:635–639.

20 Torres AJ, Landa JI, Moreno-Azcoita M, Arguello JM, Silecchia G, Castro J, Hernandez-Merlo F, Jover JM, Moreno-Gonzales E, Balibrea JL: Somatostatin in the management of gastrointestinal fistulas. A multicenter trial. Arch Surg 1992;127:97–99.

21 Hernandez-Aranda JC, Gallo-Chico B, Flores-Ramirez LA, Avalos-Huante R, Magos-Vazquez FJ, Ramirez-Barba EJ: Treatment of enterocutaneous fistula with or without octreotide and parenteral nutrition. Nutr Hosp 1996;11: 226–229.

22 Scott NA, Finnegan S, Irving MH: Octreotide and postoperative enterocutaneous fistulae: A controlled prospective study. Acta Gastroenterol Belg 1993;56:266–270.

23 Sancho JJ, di Costanzo J, Nubiola P, Larrad A, Beguiristain A, Roqueta F, Franch G, Oliva A, Gubern JM, Sitges-Serra A: Randomized double-blind placebo-controlled trial of early octreotide in patients with postoperative enterocutaneous fistula. Br J Surg 1995;82:638–641.

Digestion

Digestion 1999;60(suppl 2):57

Outlook

The discovery of hypothalamic factors that inhibit growth hormone secretion and of pancreatic factors that inhibit insulin secretion were the first clues to the existence of somatostatin. With the isolation and chemical characterization of somatostatin, and the availability of large amounts of peptide, it was possible to unravel the physiological functions of somatostatin. Subsequent work revealed that somatostatin was part of a multigene family, with tissue-specific processing. Many of the details of biosynthesis and genetic control have been worked out. The development of synthetic analogues such as octreotide with improved kinetic properties has made it possible to treat different endocrine and gastrointestinal diseases. The chapters of this supplement have focused on the efficacy of octreotide in managing gastrointestinal disorders. Data are presented showing that octreotide is helpful in suppressing symptoms in neuroendocrine gut tumors; evidence has been provided that octreotide reduces postsurgical complications in patients undergoing pancreatic resections; octreotide seems to be helpful in patients with noninfectious secretory diarrhea and there is recent information that acute variceal bleeding can be controlled with octreotide. The effect of octreotide in nonvariceal hemorrhage is less clear and additional studies are required to document a significant effect.

Where do we go from here? First, an application of octreotide, especially in the form of octreotide LAR®, can be envisaged in the long-term management of portal hypertension. Although endoscopic procedures are widely used to prevent or reduce recurrent hemorrhage, rebleeding occurs in approximately 30% of patients before variceal obliteration is achieved. The results of a preliminary trial suggest that octreotide may indeed be valuable in the long-term management of portal hypertension; these results, although encouraging, require additional data in form of randomized, controlled studies to establish a role for this compound in this indication. It is even conceivable that octreotide could be used in the primary prevention of variceal bleeding in patients with portal hypertension in an attempt to improve survival in these patients. No information is currently available to support this indication.

A second new application for octreotide could be the use of octreotide LAR® in the treatment of certain tumors. Preliminary data have suggested that octreotide improves the survival of patients with advanced hepatocellular carcinoma. As no specific treatment is available in these patients, octreotide offers new hope. A large, randomized, controlled trial is necessary to confirm the efficacy of the compound in these patients.

Finally, somatostatin has been shown to inhibit a variety of hormones and growth factors. Some of these factors have been implicated in the pathogenesis of angiopathy in patients with diabetes mellitus. Administration of octreotide LAR® in patients with insulin-dependent diabetes could be helpful to retard or even prevent the development of angiopathy. It is too early to speculate on this indication, but it is clear that the new form of octreotide offers new opportunites which should capture the excitement of every researcher and clinician.

Basel, February 1999 *Ch. Beglinger*

KARGER

Fax + 41 61 306 12 34
E-Mail karger@karger.ch
www.karger.ch

0012–2823/99/0608–0057$17.50/0

Accessible online at:
http//BioMedNet.com/karger

Digestion

Author Index Vol. 60, Suppl. 2, 1999

Subject Index Vol. 60, Suppl. 2, 1999

KARGER

Fax +41 61 306 12 34
E-Mail karger@karger.ch
www.karger.ch

Accessible online at:
http//BioMedNet.com/karger

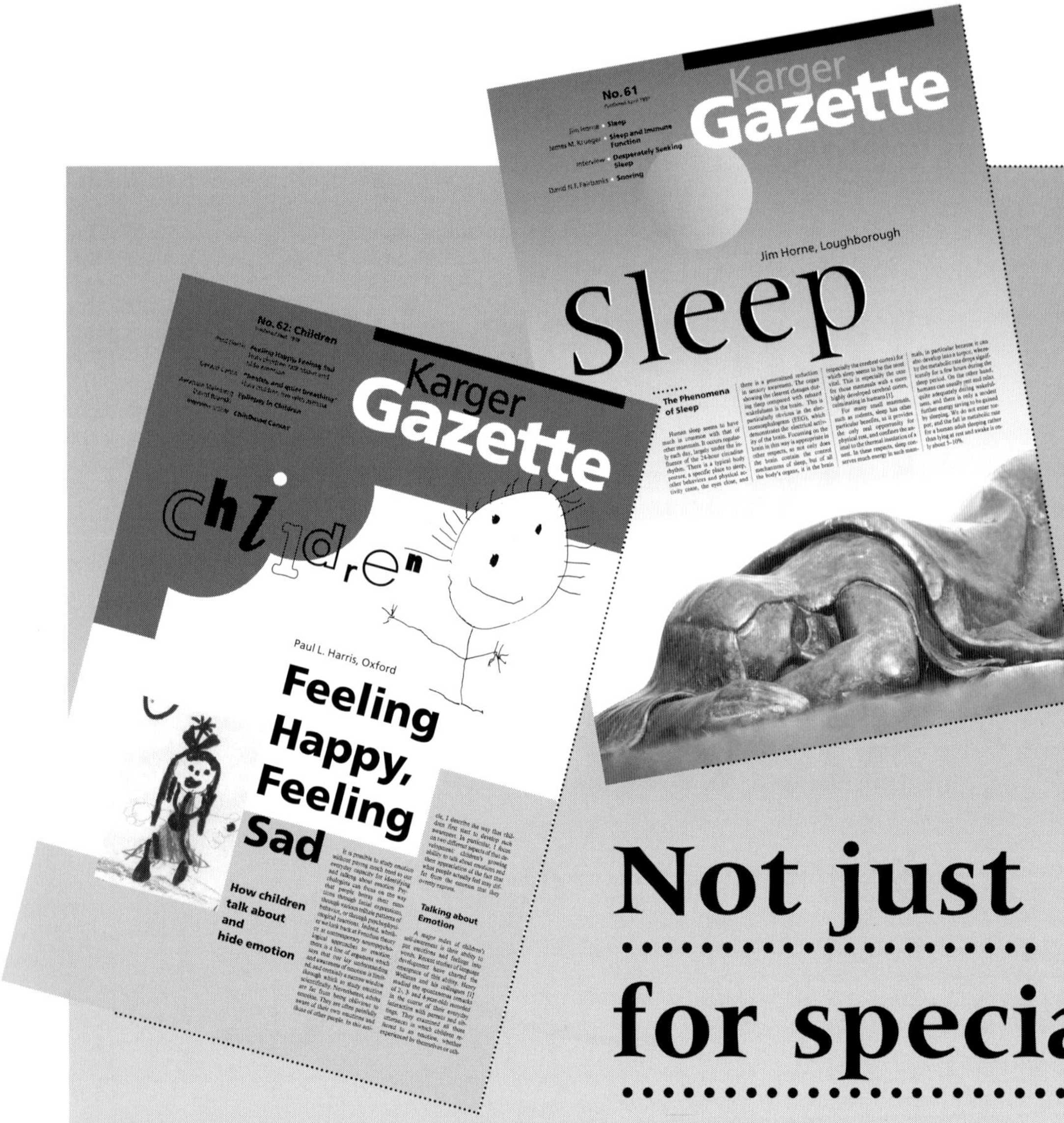

Not just for specialists

The biomedical themes of the *Karger Gazette* are topical, urgent, exciting. Its articles, written by experts from all over the world, provide a wide audience with the basic issues, new findings and controversies in a lively and readable style. Alongside invited contributions, each number carries attractively presented support material, such as informative graphics, historical summaries, interviews, and portraits of individuals and institutions. The *Karger Gazette* appears once a year. And what's more – it's free. To see behind the cover, please write, fax or e-mail us, and we'll start your subscription with the latest issue.

KARGER

S. Karger AG
Karger Gazette
P.O. Box
CH–4009 Basel (Switzerland)
Fax +41 61 306 12 34
E-Mail karger@karger.ch
www.karger.com

KI 98301